D0217563

Ultrasound Scanning:
Principles
and Protocols

Ultrasound Scanning: Principles and Protocols

Betty Bates Tempkin, BA, RT(R), RDMS

W.B. SAUNDERS COMPANY
Harcourt Brace Jovanovich, Inc.
Philadelphia   London   Toronto   Montreal   Sydney   Tokyo

W.B. SAUNDERS COMPANY
Harcourt Brace Jovanovich, Inc.

The Curtis Center
Independence Square West
Philadelphia, Pennsylvania 19106

Library of Congress Cataloging-in-Publication Data

Tempkin, Betty Bates.

   Ultrasound scanning : principles and protocols : pathology, aorta, IVC, abdomen, gynecology, obstetrics, prostate, small parts, and vascular procedures / Betty Bates Tempkin ; contributing authors, Kristin Dykstra-Downey, Felicia M. Terry.

     p. cm.
   ISBN 0-7216-3706-X

   1. Diagnosis, Ultrasonic. I. Dykstra-Downey, Kristin. II. Terry, Felicia M.
III. Title.
    [DNLM: 1. Clinical Protocols. 2. Ultrasonography—methods. 3. Ultrasonography—standards. WB 289 T283u]

  RC78.7.U4T46 1993

  616.07′543—dc20

  DNLM/DLC   91-35981

Ultrasound Scanning: Principles and Protocols   ISBN 0-7216-3706-X

Copyright © 1993 by W. B. Saunders Company

All rights reserved. No part of this publication may be reproduced or transmitted in any form or by any means, electronic or mechanical, including photocopy, recording, or any information storage and retrieval system, without permission in writing from the publisher.

Printed in Mexico.

Last digit is the print number: 9   8   7   6   5   4   3   2   1

To David,
who enhances every part of my life
and to my parents,
Bates and Esther Pauley,
who have given me the foundation
upon which this book and many successes have been built.

BBT

CONTRIBUTORS

KRISTIN DYKSTRA-DOWNEY, AAS, RT(R), ARDMS
Applications Specialist, Acoustic Imaging, Phoenix, Arizona;
formerly Professor and Director of Diagnostic Medical
Sonography Program, Hillsborough Community College,
Tampa, Florida
Neonatal Brain Scanning Protocol

FELICIA M. TERRY, AS, BS, RDMS, RVT
Program Director, Ultrasound, Tidewater Community
College, Virginia Beach, Virginia
*Abdominal Doppler and Color Flow; Duplex Carotid Artery
Scanning Protocol; Peripheral Vascular Scanning Protocols*

PREFACE

Ultrasound Scanning Principles and Protocols came about as a result of my teaching and practical scanning experience.

During my ten years as a sonographer—most of which I have spent teaching sonography students in scanning labs as well as in the hospital setting—I realized that student sonographers needed a basic approach to the performance of scans, a pattern as well as a benchmark for their work. My purpose in writing this text is to provide a step-by-step method for scanning and image documentation because it should be the sonographer's first priority to provide appropriate images for physician interpretation. It is my hope that this "how to" scanning approach will take the struggle out of scanning while ensuring thoroughness and accuracy. By enumerating scanning principles and providing complete documentation of each examination, I hope to ensure scanning standardization and to improve exam quality.

This book is structured so as to be easy to read, simple to follow, and practical to use. The text covers scanning protocols for abdominal vasculature (aorta, IVC) and abdominal organs (liver, gallbladder and biliary tract, pancreas, kidneys, spleen). Pelvic scanning protocols include the female pelvis (gyn, endovaginal), obstetrics, and the male pelvis (prostate, endorectal). Small parts protocols cover the thyroid, scrotum, breast, popliteal artery, and neonatal brain. In addition, vascular scanning protocols include abdominal Doppler and color flow analysis, duplex carotid artery scanning, and peripheral vascular scanning.

Throughout this book I have provided criteria and specifics for scanning and documenting pathology and have also addressed professionalism, clinical skills, equipment, film labeling, technique, and film-case presentation. Technical parameters that include scanning planes and their interpretation, transducer positions, patient positions, and defining long axis are also included in the text. Each protocol chapter selectively discusses location, anatomy, physiology, sonographic appearance, normal variants, patient preparation, transducer placement, breathing technique, longitudinal survey, transverse survey, and required pictures. Scanning topics contain survey reference illustrations. Each required sonographic image is accompanied by a schematic of that image. Although I have assumed that the reader has a working knowledge of gross and sectional anatomy, each chapter begins with an overview of anatomy and reference illustrations.

I have used only up-to-date images from state-of-the-art equipment. Applicable scanning protocols follow the American Institute of Ultrasound in Medicine guidelines, which are included in the appendices at the end of this book (along with an abbreviations glossary) to assist the reader. Since this text represents my personal experience in scanning and teaching, the chapters highlight scanning methods that I have found to work best. But the beauty of ultrasound scanning is its total dependence on operator skill, and thus multiple approaches to solving imaging problems are not only expected but unavoidable. Therefore, in addition to my favorite ways of doing things, I have also given alternatives, and I encourage you to explore other approaches.

What makes the sonographer's role in medicine unique from those of other allied health professionals is the total dependence on the skill of the operator. When performed at the highest level, the sonographer's contribution is an integral part of patient evaluation. It is my hope that this text will contribute directly to the achievement of excellence in the daily practice of sonography.

BETTY BATES TEMPKIN, BA, RT(R), RDMS

ACKNOWLEDGMENTS

It is with much pleasure that I have this opportunity to thank the people that have been instrumental in my sonography career and in the making of this book.

I have been fortunate to have reaped the benefits of wisdom from the following people: Magdalena Pogonowska, MD, Marie Mandelstamm, MD, Donna Ingram, RDMS, Carol Mittelstaedt, MD, Eric Rosenberg, MD, and Jim Bowie, MD. Thank you for your guidance and inspiration.

A special thank you to my contributors and dear friends, Kristin Dykstra-Downey, AS, RT(R), RDMS, and Felicia M. Terry, AS, BS, RDMS, RVT. It is always a pleasure!

Further, an acknowledgment to all of my students whose desire and interest brought this project about. I particularly want to thank two former students, Brenda K. Sandridge, RT(R), RDMS, who is responsible for the obstetrical images in the book, and Katherine Hall, AS, RT(R), RDMS, who volunteered to be scanned for some of those images. Currently, they are both staff sonographers at Duke University Medical Center.

In addition, thank you Nell Strickland, RT(R), RDMS, also a Duke University Medical Center sonographer, who not only contributed to my early scanning career but also provided the scrotum images.

Many thanks to Debbie Wernerberger, BS, RDMS, sonographer and lecturer at Thomas Jefferson University Sonography Program, for providing the endovaginal images, and to the sonography staff at The Methodist Hospital in Houston, Texas for the endorectal images.

Thanks also to those who volunteered to be scanned, especially former student and staff sonographer Beth Kline, RDMS. Thanks to them, Kay Ballard and Dupont Film, and the Acoustic Imaging System, the abdomen, gyn, thyroid, and popliteal images turned out beautifully!

I also want my husband, David Tempkin, MD, to know how much I appreciate his encouragement, expertise as a sonologist, and unique style!

A special acknowledgment to the American Institute of Ultrasound in Medicine and Kathleen M. Wilson, Director of Publications, for agreeing to include the AIUM scanning guidelines in the book. I feel that this collaboration will greatly benefit the reader and ultimately the ultrasound community.

I am especially grateful to Earle Pitts and York Graphic Services, Inc., for their contribution in bringing my ideas to life with their exceptional art work.

And finally, but very importantly, a heartfelt thanks to my editor, Lisa Biello, and everyone involved with this book at the W.B. Saunders Company. Lisa Biello's interest, enthusiasm, and insight do great service to the field of sonography and made this the most pleasurable experience of my career.

BETTY BATES TEMPKIN, BA, RT(R), RDMS

CONTENTS

PART V
VASCULAR SCANNING PROTOCOLS

PART I

GENERAL
PRINCIPLES

CHAPTER ONE
INTRODUCTION

PURPOSE

- To provide a practical text with a simplified and standardized scanning protocol.
- To provide a scanning protocol that requires thoroughness.
- To provide a scanning protocol that requires appropriate images for diagnosis.

STANDARDS

- Scanning surveys in two scanning planes prior to taking images. This complete survey is the most important element of the examination because it is when the following determinations are made:
  - Correct technique.
  - Presence or lack of pathology.
  - Normal variants.
  - Image sequence.
- Surveys include:
  - Entire abdomen for abdominal organ examinations—no single-organ exams.
  - Entire pelvis.
  - Single vessels.
  - Individual small part organs.
- All film images in two scanning planes.

PROFESSIONALISM

- Practice courteous and respectful interaction with patients and staff.
- Introduce yourself to patients.
- Conversations with patients should be appropriate and professional.
- Dress appropriately and wear an identification badge.
- **Unless you are a physician, do not give patients a diagnosis.**

CLINICAL SKILLS

- Make sure you have the correct patient.
  - Check patient identification bracelet.
  - Check patient chart.
- Assist patients to and from the exam area.
- Briefly explain the examination and instruct the patient appropriately.
- Handle medical equipment attached to the patient in a safe manner.
- Assist patient in dressing in a gown when required.
- Drape patient properly.

EQUIPMENT

- Select the proper transducer for the examination.
- Be able to attach and detach transducers from the machine.
- Experiment with controls for the best image.
- Be able to load and unload film cassettes.
- Be able to set and operate the camera.

FILM LABELING

- Patient's name.
- Patient's identification number.
- Date.
- Scanning site.
- Initials of person scanning.
- Transducer megahertz.
- Area of interest.
  - Broad and specific.
  - Example: Aorta (broad) and bifurcation (specific).
- Scanning plane.
  - Sagittal.
  - Transverse.
  - Coronal.

NOTE: If an endovaginal or endorectal examination is performed, a health professional (e.g., another sonographer, nurse, physician) should witness the procedure, and his or her initials should also go on the film.

- Patient position.
  - Supine.
  - Prone.
  - Sitting erect/semierect.
  - Right lateral decubitus (RLD).
  - Left lateral decubitus (LLD).
  - Right posterior oblique (RPO).
  - Left posterior oblique (LPO).

NOTE: Film labeling should be confined to the margins surrounding the image. Never label over any part of the image unless you include the same image without the labels.

TECHNIQUE

NOTE: The following conditions should be optimal:

- Field size.
- Near gain.
- Far gain.
- Homogeneous technique from near to far field.
- Contrast.
- Well-defined borders.
- No areas of fade-out.
- Low power setting with adjusted slope (TGC).
- **Overall interpretable images.**

FILM/CASE PRESENTATION

- State exam and reason for it.
- Present patient history.
- Present patient lab data and other known correlative data such as reports and films from other imaging modalities.
- Present films in a logical sequence.
- Be able to discuss and justify techniques and procedures used.
- Be able to discuss related anatomy and pathology findings.

CHAPTER TWO
SCANNING PLANES AND
METHODS

SCANNING PLANES

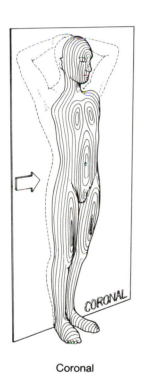

Coronal

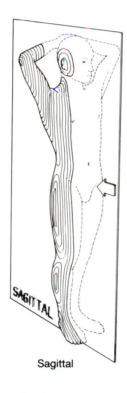

Sagittal

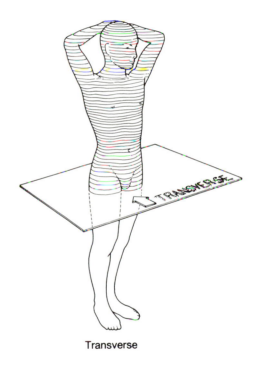

Transverse

- How ultrasound images the body.

- Two-dimensional.

- Include:
  - Sagittal planes—divide the body into unequal right and left sections parallel to the long axis of the body.

  - Transverse planes—divide the body into unequal superior and inferior sections perpendicular to the long axis of the body.

  - Coronal planes—divide the body into unequal anterior and posterior sections perpendicular to sagittal planes and parallel to the long axis of the body.

● Anatomical specifics of a sagittal plane.
Anterior or posterior approach:

- Anterior.

- Posterior.

- Superior.

- Inferior.

NOTE: Since we do not appreciate right lateral and left lateral on a sagittal scan, the transducer must be moved to the right or left of a sagittal plane to visualize adjacent anatomy.

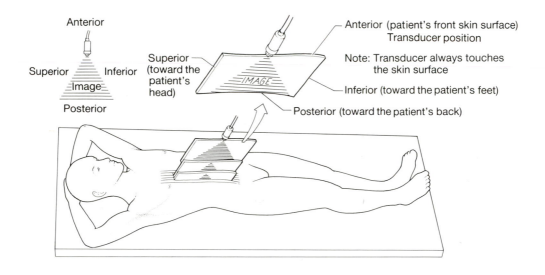

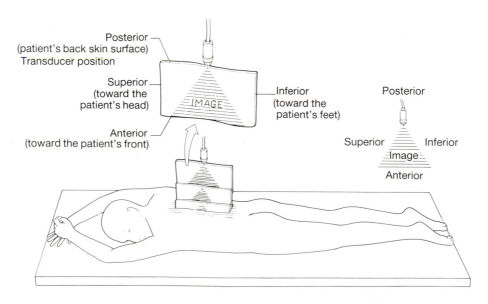

● Anatomical specifics of a transverse plane.
Anterior or posterior approach:

– Anterior.

– Posterior.

– Right lateral.

– Left lateral.

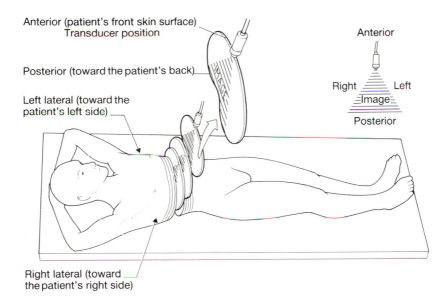

Anterior (patient's front skin surface)
Transducer position

Posterior (toward the patient's back)

Left lateral (toward the
patient's left side)

Anterior

Right   Left
Image
Posterior

Right lateral (toward
the patient's right side)

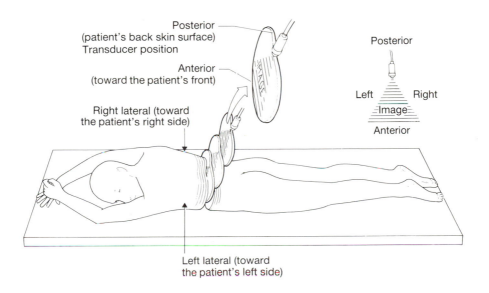

Posterior
(patient's back skin surface)
Transducer position

Anterior
(toward the patient's front)

Right lateral (toward
the patient's right side)

Posterior

Left   Right
Image
Anterior

Left lateral (toward
the patient's left side)

Right or left lateral approach:

- Lateral (right or left).
- Anterior.
- Medial.
- Posterior.

NOTE: Since we do not appreciate superior and inferior on a transverse scan, the transducer must be moved superiorly and inferiorly from a transverse plane to visualize adjacent anatomy.

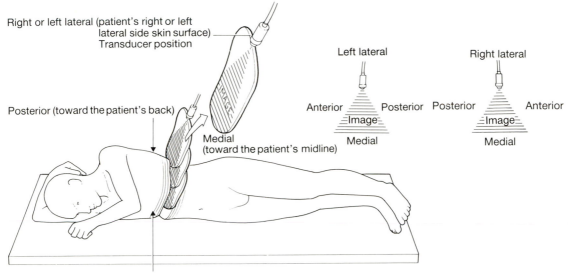

- Anatomical specifics of a coronal plane. Right or left lateral approach:
  - Lateral (right or left).
  - Superior.
  - Medial.
  - Inferior.

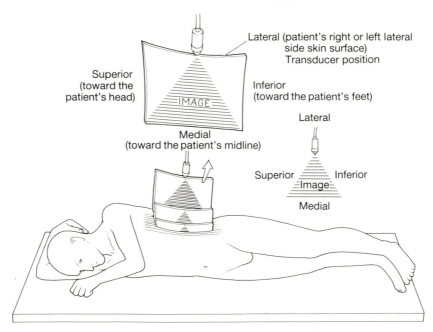

NOTE: Since we do not appreciate anterior and posterior on a coronal scan, the transducer must be moved anteriorly and posteriorly from a coronal plane to visualize adjacent anatomy.

Scanning Methods

- Organ-oriented.
    - Scan according to the lie of the organ.
    - Scanning plane may therefore be oblique.

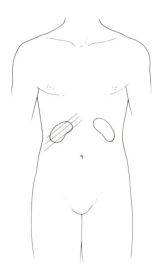

Oblique sagittals
to visualize the
longitudinal and
long axis of the
kidney

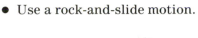

- Use a rock-and-slide motion.

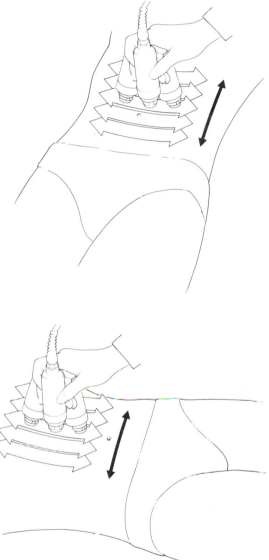

- Transducer positions.

  - Perpendicular.
    The transducer is straight up and down.

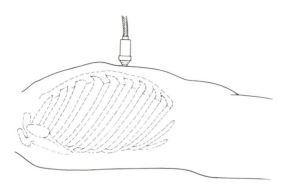

  - Intercostal.
    The transducer is between the ribs. It can be perpendicular, subcostal, or angled.

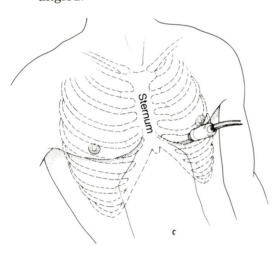

  - Rotated.
    The transducer is rotated varying degrees to oblique the scanning plane.

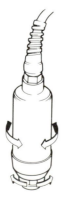

  - Subcostal.
    The transducer is angled superiorly just beneath the inferior costal margin.

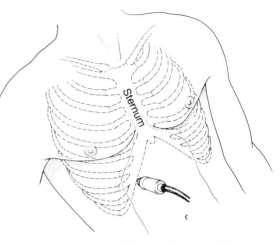

  - Angled.
    The transducer is angled superiorly, inferiorly, or right and left laterally at varying degrees.

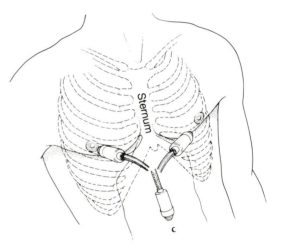

● Scanning the longitudinal of something shows its length. Scanning the long axis of something shows its longest length. The long axis of an organ or vessel can be seen in any scanning plane depending on its lie. Examples:

– Abdominal aorta:
   Lies superior to inferior in the body. Longitudinal and long axes seen in the sagittal and coronal scanning planes.

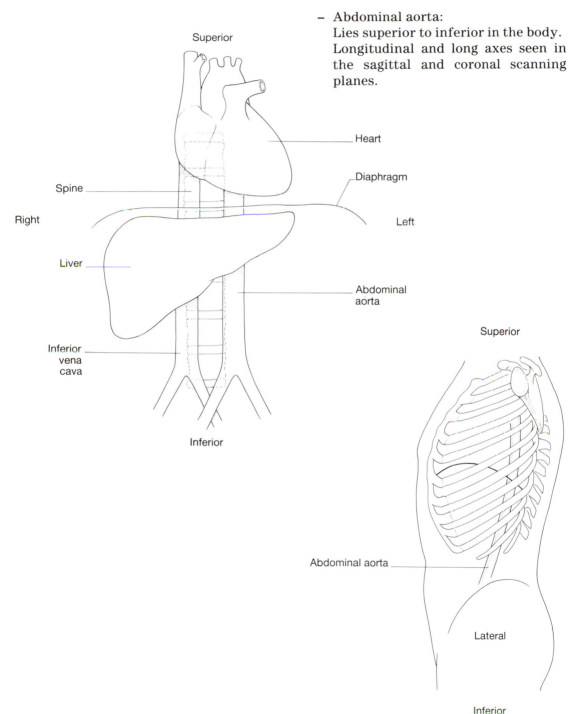

– Gallbladder:
   Lie is variable. Can lie superior to inferior or right to left.

– Longitudinal and long axes seen in the sagittal and coronal scanning planes when lying superior to inferior.
   Longitudinal and long axes seen in the transverse scanning plane when lying right to left.

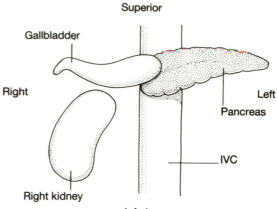

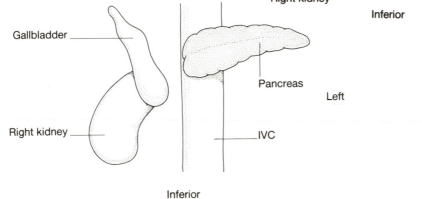

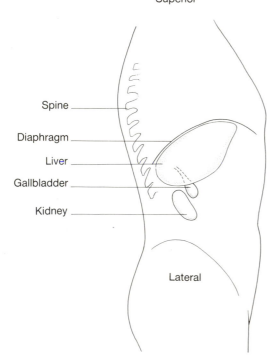

- Patient positions.

  - Supine.
    The patient lies on his or her back.

  - Prone.
    The patient lies on his or her front.

  - Sitting erect/semierect.

  - Right lateral decubitus (RLD).
    The patient lies on his or her right side with the left arm up over the head.

  - Left lateral decubitus (LLD).
    The patient lies on his or her left side with the right arm up over the head.

  - Right posterior oblique (RPO).
    The patient lies on his or her back with the left side of the body elevated at a 45-degree angle.

  - Left posterior oblique (LPO).
    The patient lies on his or her back with the right side of the body elevated at a 45-degree angle.

NOTE: Patient position should not be changed while taking images of an organ unless predetermined during the survey or out of necessity because of gas obliteration.

- Follow the scanning protocols.

- Anatomical scanning reference:

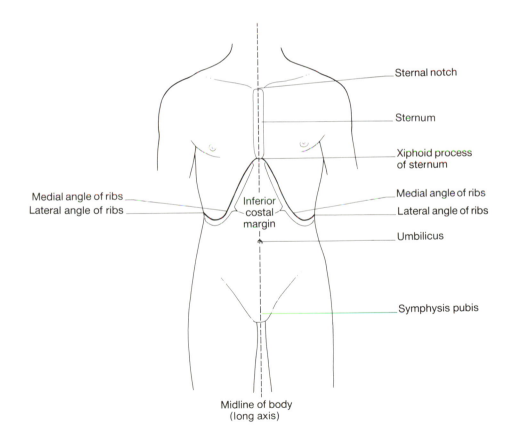

Sternal notch

Sternum

Xiphoid process of sternum

Medial angle of ribs
Lateral angle of ribs

Inferior costal margin

Medial angle of ribs
Lateral angle of ribs

Umbilicus

Symphysis pubis

Midline of body
(long axis)

CHAPTER THREE
PATHOLOGY SCANNING
PROTOCOL

CRITERIA

- Survey in at least two scanning planes.
- Volume measurements.
- High- and low-gain images in two scanning planes.

SURVEY

- In at least two scanning planes.
- To follow survey of primary organ(s) or vessel(s).
- Manipulate technique (high- to low-gain settings) to determine composition.

REQUIRED PICTURES

NOTE: Required pictures of pathology follow the required pictures of the primary organ(s) or vessel(s).

1. LONGITUDINAL IMAGE WITH *MEASUREMENT FROM MOST SUPERIOR TO MOST INFERIOR MARGIN.*
   LABELED: "PRIMARY ORGAN" OR "SITE" (ADJACENT ORGAN[S]) "SCANNING PLANE"

NOTE: It may be difficult to define the primary organ of pathology. If so, the site and adjacent organs must be noted and labeled. Look for echogenic interfaces where fat separates adjacent structures.

2. SAME IMAGE AS NUMBER 1 WITHOUT CALIPERS.
3. TRANSVERSE IMAGE WITH *MEASUREMENTS FROM ANTERIOR TO POSTERIOR AND LATERAL TO LATERAL OR LATERAL TO MEDIAL AT LARGEST DIMENSIONS.*
   LABELED: "PRIMARY ORGAN" OR "SITE" (ADJACENT ORGAN[S]) "SCANNING PLANE"

4. SAME IMAGE AS NUMBER 3 WITHOUT CALIPERS.

5. LONGITUDINAL IMAGE AT HIGH GAIN.
   LABELED: "PRIMARY ORGAN" OR "SITE" (ADJACENT ORGAN[S]) "SCANNING PLANE"

6. TRANSVERSE IMAGE AT HIGH GAIN.
   LABELED: "PRIMARY ORGAN" OR "SITE" (ADJACENT ORGAN[S]) "SCANNING PLANE"

7. LONGITUDINAL IMAGE AT LOW GAIN.

LABELED: "PRIMARY ORGAN" OR "SITE" (ADJACENT ORGAN[S]) "SCANNING PLANE"

8. TRANSVERSE IMAGE AT LOW GAIN.

LABELED: "PRIMARY ORGAN" OR "SITE" (ADJACENT ORGAN[S]) "SCANNING PLANE"

NOTE: Depending on the site and complexity of the pathology, additional images (in at least two scanning planes) may be necessary. Example: If a localized area is partially solid and partially necrotic, and both areas cannot be visualized on the same image, both areas must be filmed separately in two scanning planes.

PART II

ABDOMINAL SCANNING PROTOCOLS

CHAPTER FOUR

Abdominal Scanning Protocols: Overview

STANDARD

- No single-organ examinations.
- Images vary according to whether or not an organ is the primary area of emphasis.
- Protocols give image specifics.
- Use real-time scanners with sector or curved linear transducers.

SURVEY

- Exams begin with a survey of abdominal organs and major vessels or specific vessel in two scanning planes.
- Abdominal organ surveys begin at the aorta to be followed by the other organs in any sequence you choose. Suggest liver and IVC followed by biliary system, pancreas, right kidney, left kidney, and spleen.
- Protocols give survey specifications.
- Surveys do not vary. Organ surveys are the same whether or not an organ is the primary area of emphasis.
- Do not interrupt one survey with another.
- Do not take any images during the survey. The survey is used to determine the correct technique, presence or lack of pathology, recognition of any normal variants, and the sequence in which you will take images.

- If pathology is seen, it is surveyed after the primary organ(s) or vessel(s) in two scanning planes.

CONSIDERATIONS

- Sonographic patterns in the abdomen:
  - Organs, muscles, and tissues: echo texture.
  - Blood vessels and ducts: anechoic lumens, echogenic walls.
  - GI tract: hypoechoic walls, varying degrees of echogenic (gas) to hypoechoic (fluid) centers.
  - Bone: echogenic.
- Echo texture of abdominal organs should be homogeneous. Note that this parenchymal pattern changes with disease processes.
- Experiment using different amounts of transducer pressure on the skin surface. More often than not you can press the transducer harder than you realize and, in turn, improve image quality. Always make sure that the patient is comfortable.

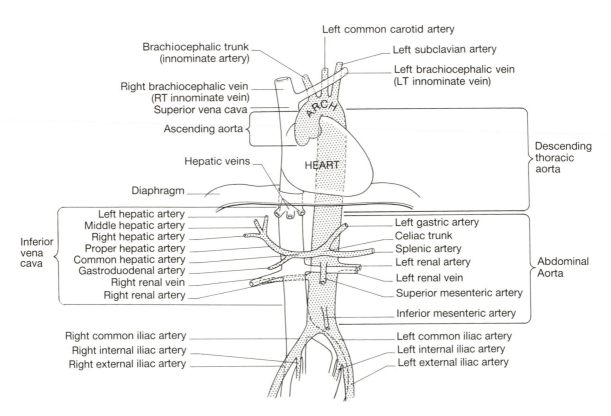

Left common carotid artery

Brachiocephalic trunk (innominate artery)

Left subclavian artery

Left brachiocephalic vein (LT innominate vein)

Right brachiocephalic vein (RT innominate vein)

Superior vena cava

Ascending aorta

Descending thoracic aorta

Hepatic veins

Diaphragm

Left hepatic artery

Middle hepatic artery

Right hepatic artery

Proper hepatic artery

Common hepatic artery

Gastroduodenal artery

Right renal vein

Right renal artery

Left gastric artery

Celiac trunk

Splenic artery

Left renal artery

Left renal vein

Superior mesenteric artery

Inferior mesenteric artery

Inferior vena cava

Abdominal Aorta

Right common iliac artery

Right internal iliac artery

Right external iliac artery

Left common iliac artery

Left internal iliac artery

Left external iliac artery

Location and anatomy of the aorta

ABDOMINAL VASCULATURE

CHAPTER FIVE
ABDOMINAL AORTA SCANNING PROTOCOL

LOCATION

- Originates at the left ventricle.

- Ascends posterior to the pulmonary artery.

- Arches to the left.

- Descends (thoracic aorta) posterior to the diaphragm into the retroperitoneum of the abdominal cavity (abdominal aorta).

- Descends anterior to the spine to the left of the inferior vena cava.

- Bifurcates into the common iliac arteries anterior to the body of the fourth lumbar vertebra.

ANATOMY

- Consists of three muscle layers:
  - Intima (innermost).
  - Media (middle layer).
  - Adventitia (outer).

- Largest artery in the body.

- Branches:
  - Celiac trunk (branches into the left gastric artery, hepatic artery, and splenic artery).
  - Superior mesenteric artery (SMA).
  - Inferior mesenteric artery (IMA).
  - Renal arteries.

- Size is normal up to 3 cm in diameter gradually tapering toward the bifurcation.

- Can be very tortuous.

PHYSIOLOGY

- Supplies the organs, bones, and connective structures of the body with oxygen and nutrient-rich blood.

SONOGRAPHIC APPEARANCE

- Echogenic muscular walls.
- Anechoic, echo-free lumen.

PATIENT PREP

- Fasting for at least 8 hours.
- If the patient has eaten, still attempt the examination.

PATIENT POSITION

- **Supine, right lateral decubitus.**
- Left lateral decubitus, left posterior oblique, right posterior oblique, or sitting semierect to erect as needed.

NOTE: Different patient positions should be used whenever the suggested position does not give the desired results.

TRANSDUCER

- **3.0 MHz** or **3.5 MHz.**
- 5.0 MHz for thin patients.

BREATHING TECHNIQUE

- **Normal respiration.**
- Deep, held respiration.

NOTE: Different breathing techniques should be used whenever the suggested breathing technique does not give the desired results.

AORTA SURVEY

NOTE: While surveying the aorta, evaluate the periaortic regions for adenopathy.

LONGITUDINAL SURVEY

Sagittal Plane/Anterior Approach

● BEGIN WITH THE TRANSDUCER PERPENDICULAR, AT THE MIDLINE OF THE BODY, JUST INFERIOR TO THE XIPHOID PROCESS OF THE STERNUM.

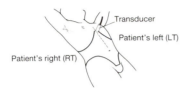

Transducer
Patient's left (LT)
Patient's right (RT)

● MOVE OR ANGLE THE TRANSDUCER TO THE PATIENT'S RIGHT AND IDENTIFY THE DISTAL IVC POSTERIOR TO THE LIVER.

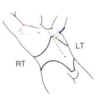

LT
RT

● MOVE OR ANGLE THE TRANSDUCER TO THE PATIENT'S LEFT AND IDENTIFY THE PROXIMAL AORTA POSTERIOR TO THE LIVER.

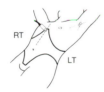

RT
LT

N O T E: The aorta is posterior to the diaphragm. The IVC passes through the diaphragm.

● WHILE VIEWING THE PROXIMAL AORTA, SLOWLY MOVE INFERIORLY, USING A ROCK-AND-SLIDE MOTION. SLIGHTLY ROCK RIGHT TO LEFT TO SCAN THROUGH EACH SIDE OF THE AORTA WHILE SLIDING INFERIORLY. IT MAY BE NECESSARY TO ROTATE THE TRANSDUCER AT VARYING DEGREES (TO OBLIQUE THE SCANNING PLANE ACCORDING TO THE LIE OF THE AORTA) TO VISUALIZE THE LONG AXIS OF THE AORTA. NOTE AND EVALUATE THE ANTERIOR BRANCHES: CELIAC, SMA.

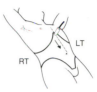

LT
RT

● CONTINUE ROCKING AND SLIDING THE TRANSDUCER INFERIORLY THROUGH THE MIDDLE AND DISTAL AORTA TO THE BIFURCATION (USUALLY AT OR JUST BEYOND THE LEVEL OF THE UMBILICUS).

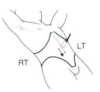

LT
RT

N O T E : The longitudinal of the bifurcation can be difficult to visualize in the sagittal plane. Visualization can be easier from the coronal plane.

Sagittal Plane/Anterior Approach

- Patient **supine**, left posterior oblique, right posterior oblique, or sitting semierect to erect.

- From the lateral aspects of the most distal aorta, angle the transducer back toward the aorta and slightly move inferiorly until the bifurcation and common iliac arteries are seen.

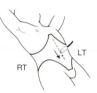

Coronal Plane/Left Lateral Approach

- Patient **right lateral decubitus**, supine, sitting semierect to erect, or left lateral decubitus.

- Begin with the transducer perpendicular, midcoronal plane, just superior to the iliac crest.

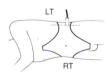

- Use the inferior pole of the left kidney as a landmark and look for the bifurcation medial and inferior.

- It may be necessary to rotate the transducer at varying degrees to visualize the long axis of the bifurcation and common iliac arteries.

N O T E : To avoid moving the patient, survey of the bifurcation in the decubitus position can be done after the transverse survey.

N O T E : While longitudinal evaluation of the proximal and middle aorta is generally easier from the sagittal plane approach, the coronal plane approach can be used. Move the transducer superiorly from the level of the bifurcation or scan intercostally, looking for the aorta medially. Label any images that follow accordingly.

TRANSVERSE SURVEY

Transverse Plane/Anterior Approach

● BEGIN WITH THE TRANSDUCER PERPENDICULAR, AT THE MIDLINE OF THE BODY, JUST INFERIOR TO THE XIPHOID PROCESS OF THE STERNUM.

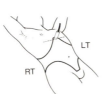

● ANGLE THE TRANSDUCER SUPERIORLY UNTIL THE HEART IS SEEN. SLOWLY, STRAIGHTENING THE TRANSDUCER TO PERPENDICULAR, LOOK FOR THE AORTA JUST TO THE LEFT OF MIDLINE. THE AORTA WILL APPEAR ROUND OR OVAL-SHAPED. ALTERNATIVELY, IN THE SAGITTAL PLANE LOCATE THE LONGITUDINAL OF THE PROXIMAL AORTA, THEN ROTATE THE TRANSDUCER 90 DEGREES INTO THE TRANSVERSE PLANE.

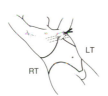

● WHILE VIEWING THE PROXIMAL AORTA, SLOWLY MOVE INFERIORLY, USING A ROCK-AND-SLIDE MOTION. SLIGHTLY ROCK SUPERIORLY TO INFERIORLY WHILE SLIDING INFERIORLY. THIS WAY YOU SHOULD NEVER LOSE SIGHT OF THE AORTA. NOTE AND EVALUATE THE ANTERIOR BRANCHES: CELIAC, SMA.

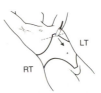

● CONTINUE ROCKING AND SLIDING THE TRANSDUCER INFERIORLY THROUGH THE MIDDLE AND DISTAL AORTA TO THE BIFURCATION. NOTE AND EVALUATE THE LATERAL BRANCHES: RENAL ARTERIES.

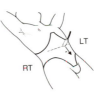

● AT THE LEVEL OF THE BIFURCATION, EVALUATE THE COMMON ILIAC ARTERIES BY SCANNING THROUGH THEM INFERIORLY UNTIL YOU LOSE SIGHT OF THEM.

Required Pictures

LONGITUDINAL IMAGES

Sagittal Plane/Anterior Approach

1. LONGITUDINAL IMAGE OF THE PROXIMAL AORTA. (INFERIOR TO THE DIAPHRAGM AND SUPERIOR TO THE CELIAC TRUNK).

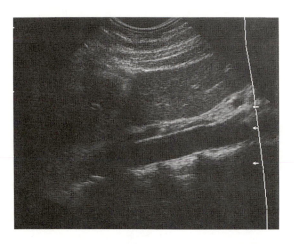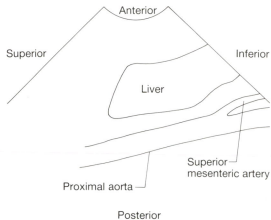

LABELED: AORTA SAG PROX

2. LONGITUDINAL IMAGE OF THE MIDDLE AORTA. (INFERIOR TO THE CELIAC TRUNK AND ALONG THE LENGTH OF THE SMA).

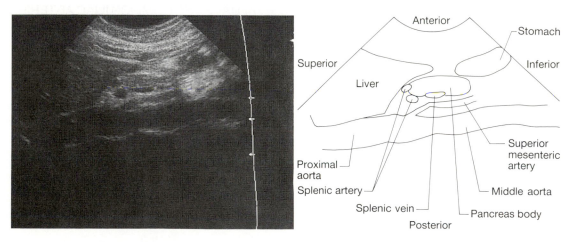

LABELED: AORTA SAG MID

3. LONGITUDINAL IMAGE OF THE DISTAL AORTA. (INFERIOR TO THE SMA AND SUPERIOR TO THE BIFURCATION).

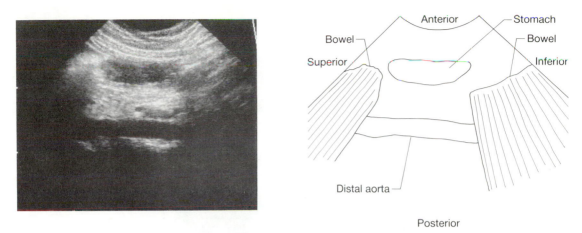

LABELED: AORTA SAG DISTAL

4. LONGITUDINAL IMAGE OF THE AORTA BIFURCATION. (COMMON ILIAC ARTERIES).

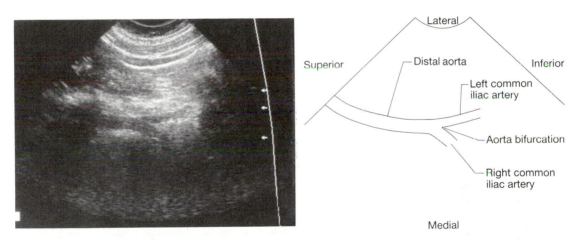

LABELED: AORTA SAG BIF RT OR LT OBL (DEPENDING ON THE LATERAL ASPECT YOU ANGLE THE TRANSDUCER FROM) OR AORTA LT OR RT COR BIF

NOTE: To avoid moving the patient, longitudinal images of the bifurcation in the decubitus position can be taken after the transverse images. Although the coronal plane approach can be used with the patient supine, the decubitus position is generally easier and can be helpful if the patient has obscuring bowel gas anteriorly.

TRANSVERSE IMAGES

Transverse Plane/Anterior Approach

5. TRANSVERSE IMAGE OF THE PROXIMAL AORTA WITH *ANTERIOR TO POSTERIOR MEASUREMENT (CALIPERS OUTSIDE WALL TO OUTSIDE WALL)*. (INFERIOR TO THE DIAPHRAGM AND SUPERIOR TO THE CELIAC TRUNK).

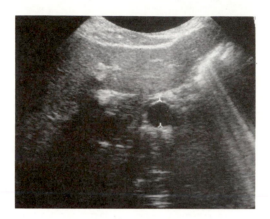

LABELED: AORTA TRV PROX

6. SAME IMAGE AS NUMBER 5 WITHOUT CALIPERS.

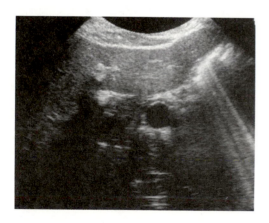 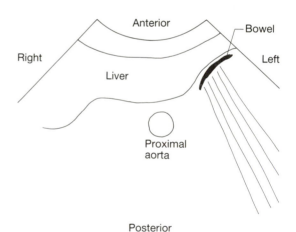

7. TRANSVERSE IMAGE OF THE MIDDLE AORTA WITH *ANTERIOR TO POSTE-RIOR MEASUREMENT (CALIPERS OUTSIDE WALL TO OUTSIDE WALL).* (INFERIOR TO THE CELIAC TRUNK, *AT THE LEVEL OF THE RENAL ARTERIES,* AND ALONG THE LENGTH OF THE SMA).

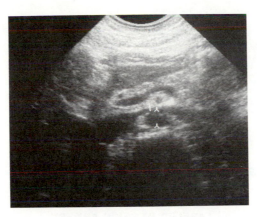

LABELED: AORTA TRV MID

8. SAME IMAGE AS NUMBER 7 WITHOUT CALIPERS.

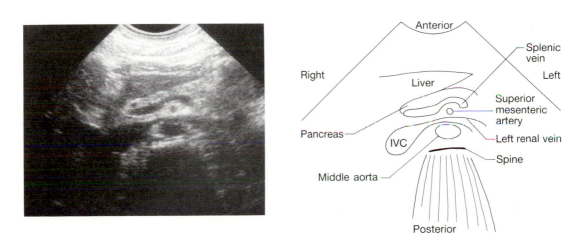

LABELED: AORTA TRV MID

NOTE: If the renal arteries are not represented on the above images, an additional image(s) of the renal arteries should be taken here and labeled accordingly.

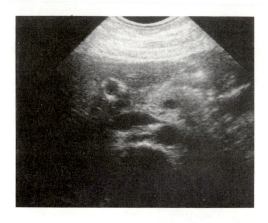
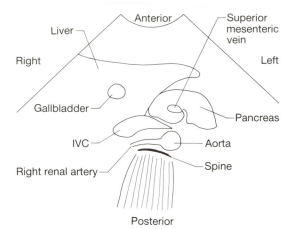

LABELED: RT RENAL ART TRV

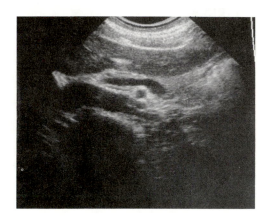
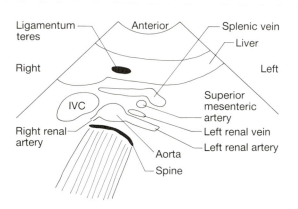

LABELED: LT: RENAL ART TRV

9. TRANSVERSE IMAGE OF THE DISTAL AORTA WITH *ANTERIOR TO POSTE-RIOR MEASUREMENT (CALIPERS OUTSIDE WALL TO OUTSIDE WALL)* (IN-FERIOR TO THE SMA AND SUPERIOR TO THE BIFURCATION).

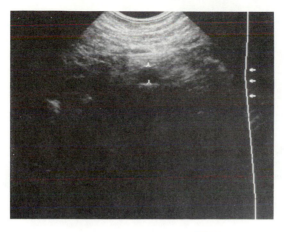

LABELED: AORTA TRV DISTAL

10. SAME IMAGE AS NUMBER 9 WITHOUT CALIPERS.

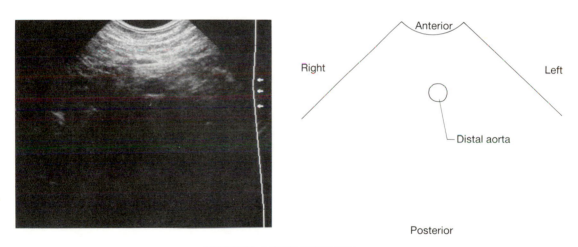

LABELED: AORTA TRV DISTAL

11. TRANSVERSE IMAGE OF THE BIFURCATION. (COMMON ILIAC ARTERIES).

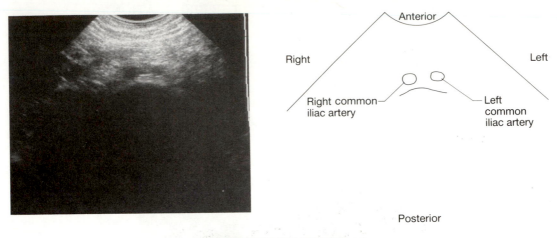

LABELED: AORTA TRV BIF

REQUIRED PICTURES WHEN THE ABDOMINAL AORTA IS NOT THE PRIMARY AREA OF INTEREST

1. LONGITUDINAL IMAGE OF THE PROXIMAL AND MIDDLE AORTA.

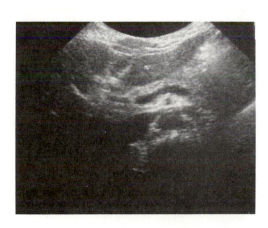
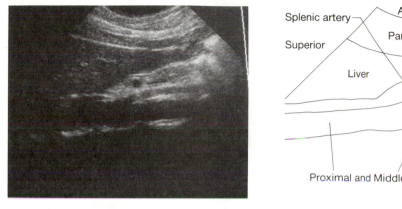

LABELED: AORTA SAG MID

2. TRANSVERSE IMAGE OF THE MIDDLE AORTA AT THE LEVEL OF THE RENAL ARTERIES.

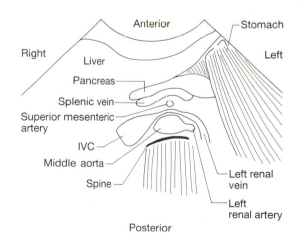
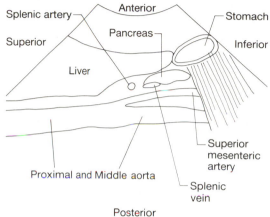

LABELED: AORTA TRV MID

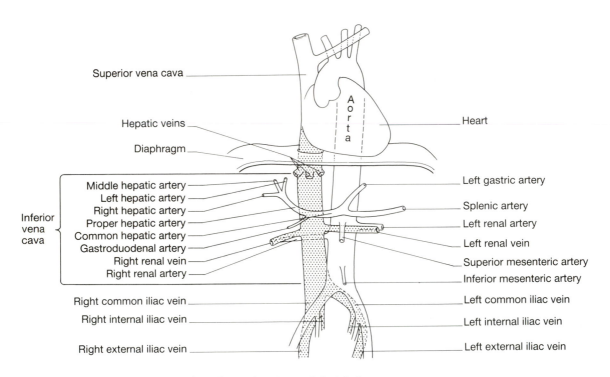

Location and anatomy of the inferior vena cava

Superior vena cava

Hepatic veins

Diaphragm

Aorta

Heart

Inferior vena cava

Middle hepatic artery
Left hepatic artery
Right hepatic artery
Proper hepatic artery
Common hepatic artery
Gastroduodenal artery
Right renal vein
Right renal artery

Left gastric artery

Splenic artery

Left renal artery

Left renal vein

Superior mesenteric artery

Inferior mesenteric artery

Right common iliac vein

Right internal iliac vein

Right external iliac vein

Left common iliac vein

Left internal iliac vein

Left external iliac vein

LOCATION

- Originates at the junction of the two common iliac veins anterior to the body of the fifth lumbar vertebra.

- Ascends the retroperitoneum of the abdominal cavity and passes through the diaphragm to enter the right atrium.

- Ascends anterior to the spine to the right of the aorta.

- Passes through a deep fossa on the posterior surface of the liver between the caudate lobe and bare area.

ANATOMY

- Consists of three muscle layers:
  - Intima (innermost).
  - Media (middle layer).
  - Adventitia (outer).
- Size is variable and normal up to 4 cm.
- Tributaries:
  - Hepatic veins.
  - Renal veins.
  - Common iliac veins.
  - Right adrenal vein.
  - Right ovarian vein or testicular vein.
  - Inferior phrenic vein.
  - Four lumbar veins.
  - Medial sacral vein.
- Can be very tortuous.

PHYSIOLOGY

- Returns deoxygenated blood from the tissues to the heart for oxygenation and recirculation.

SONOGRAPHIC APPEARANCE

- Echogenic muscular walls.
- Anechoic, echo-free lumen.

PATIENT PREP

- Fasting for at least 8 hours.
- If the patient has eaten, still attempt the examination.

PATIENT POSITION

- **Supine, left lateral decubitus.**
- Right lateral decubitus, left posterior oblique, right posterior oblique, or sitting semierect to erect as needed.

NOTE: Different patient positions should be used whenever the suggested position does not give the desired results.

TRANSDUCER

- **3.0 MHz** or **3.5 MHz.**
- 5.0 MHz for thin patients.

BREATHING TECHNIQUE

- **Normal respiration** or deep, held respiration.

NOTE: The diameter of the IVC varies depending on the level of respiration. Normal veins increase with held respiration or the Valsalva maneuver.

NOTE: Different breathing techniques should be used whenever the suggested breathing technique does not give the desired results.

INFERIOR VENA CAVA SURVEY

NOTE: While surveying the IVC evaluate the surrounding soft tissue areas for adenopathy.

LONGITUDINAL SURVEY

Sagittal Plane/Anterior Approach

● BEGIN WITH THE TRANSDUCER PER-PENDICULAR, AT THE MIDLINE OF THE BODY, JUST INFERIOR TO THE XIPHOID PROCESS OF THE STERNUM.

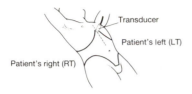

● MOVE OR ANGLE THE TRANSDUCER TO THE PATIENT'S LEFT AND IDENTIFY THE PROXIMAL AORTA POSTERIOR TO THE LIVER.

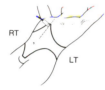

● MOVE OR ANGLE THE TRANSDUCER TO THE PATIENT'S RIGHT AND IDENTIFY THE DISTAL IVC POSTERIOR TO THE LIVER.

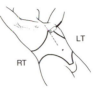

NOTE: The IVC passes through the diaphragm. The aorta passes posterior to the diaphragm.

● WHILE VIEWING THE DISTAL IVC, SLOWLY MOVE INFERIORLY, USING A ROCK-AND-SLIDE MOTION. SLIGHTLY ROCK RIGHT TO LEFT TO SCAN THROUGH EACH SIDE OF THE IVC WHILE SLIDING IN-FERIORLY. IT MAY BE NECESSARY TO RO-TATE THE TRANSDUCER AT VARYING DE-GREES (TO OBLIQUE THE SCANNING PLANE ACCORDING TO THE LIE OF THE IVC) TO VISUALIZE THE LONG AXIS OF THE IVC. NOTE AND EVALUATE THE ANTERIOR TRIBUTARIES: HEPATIC VEINS.

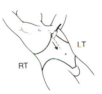

● CONTINUE ROCKING AND SLIDING THE TRANSDUCER INFERIORLY THROUGH THE MIDDLE AND PROXIMAL IVC TO THE BIFURCATION (USUALLY AT OR JUST BEYOND THE LEVEL OF THE UMBILICUS).

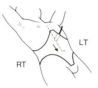

N O T E: The longitudinal of the bifurcation can be difficult to visualize in the sagittal plane. Visualization can be easier from the coronal plane:

Sagittal Plane/Anterior Approach

● Patient **supine**, left posterior oblique, right posterior oblique, or sitting semierect to erect.

● From the lateral aspects of the most proximal IVC, angle the transducer back toward the IVC and slightly move inferiorly until the bifurcation and common iliac veins are seen.

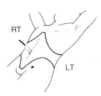

Coronal Plane/Right Lateral Approach

● Patient **left lateral decubitus**, supine, or sitting semierect to erect.

● Begin with the transducer perpendicular, midcoronal plane, just superior to the iliac crest.

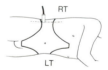

● Use the inferior pole of the right kidney as a landmark and look for the bifurcation medial and inferior.

● It may be necessary to rotate the transducer at varying degrees to visualize the long axis of the bifurcation and common iliac veins.

NOTE: To avoid moving the patient, survey of the bifurcation in the left lateral decubitus position can be done after the transverse survey.

NOTE: Although longitudinal evaluation of the distal and middle IVC is generally easier from the sagittal plane approach, the right coronal plane approach can be used. Move the transducer superiorly from the level of the bifurcation or scan intercostally, looking for the IVC medially. Label any images that follow accordingly.

TRANSVERSE SURVEY

Transverse Plane/Anterior Approach

● BEGIN WITH THE TRANSDUCER PERPENDICULAR, AT THE MIDLINE OF THE BODY, JUST INFERIOR TO THE XIPHOID PROCESS OF THE STERNUM.

● ANGLE THE TRANSDUCER SUPERIORLY UNTIL THE HEART IS SEEN. SLOWLY, STRAIGHTENING THE TRANSDUCER TO PERPENDICULAR, LOOK FOR THE IVC JUST TO THE RIGHT OF MIDLINE. THE IVC WILL APPEAR OVAL OR ALMOND-SHAPED. ALTERNATIVELY, IN THE SAGITTAL PLANE, LOCATE THE LONGITUDINAL OF THE DISTAL IVC, THEN ROTATE THE TRANSDUCER 90 DEGREES INTO THE TRANSVERSE PLANE.

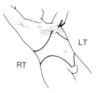

● WHILE VIEWING THE DISTAL IVC, SLOWLY MOVE INFERIORLY USING A ROCK-AND-SLIDE MOTION. SLIGHTLY ROCK SUPERIORLY TO INFERIORLY WHILE SLIDING INFERIORLY. THIS WAY YOU SHOULD NEVER LOSE SIGHT OF THE IVC. NOTE AND EVALUATE THE ANTERIOR TRIBUTARIES: HEPATIC VEINS.

● CONTINUE ROCKING AND SLIDING THE TRANSDUCER INFERIORLY THROUGH THE MIDDLE AND PROXIMAL IVC TO THE BIFURCATION. NOTE AND EVALUATE THE LATERAL TRIBUTARIES: RENAL VEINS.

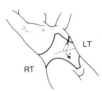

● AT THE LEVEL OF THE BIFURCATION, EVALUATE THE ILIAC VEINS BY SCANNING THROUGH THEM INFERIORLY UNTIL YOU LOSE SIGHT OF THEM.

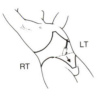

REQUIRED PICTURES

LONGITUDINAL IMAGES

Sagittal Plane/Anterior Approach

1. LONGITUDINAL IMAGE OF THE DISTAL IVC TO INCLUDE THE DIAPHRAGM AND HEPATIC VEIN(S).

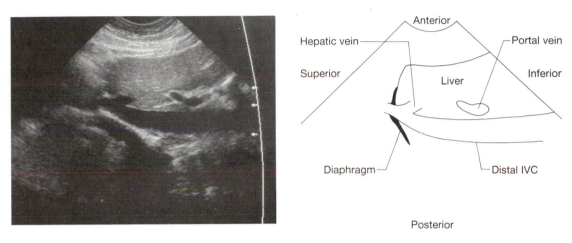

LABELED: IVC SAG DISTAL

2. LONGITUDINAL IMAGE OF THE MIDDLE IVC AT THE LEVEL OF THE HEAD OF THE PANCREAS.

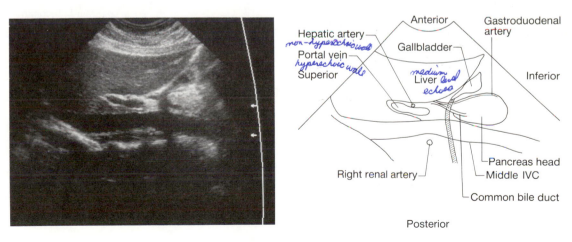

LABELED: IVC SAG MID

3. LONGITUDINAL IMAGE OF THE PROXIMAL IVC.

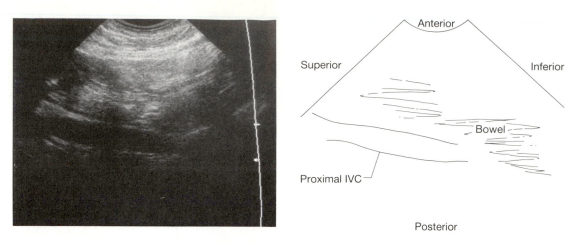

LABELED: IVC SAG PROX

4. LONGITUDINAL IMAGE OF THE IVC BIFURCATION. (COMMON ILIAC VEINS).

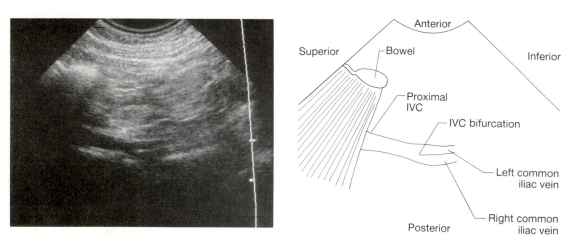

**LABELED: IVC SAG BIF RT OR LT OBL (DEPENDING ON THE LATERAL ASPECT YOU ANGLE
THE TRANSDUCER FROM) OR IVC RT COR BIF**

NOTE: To avoid moving the patient, longitudinal images of the bifurcation in the left lateral decubitus position can be taken after the transverse images. Although the coronal plane approach can be used with the patient supine, the left lateral decubitus position is generally easier and can be helpful if the patient has obscuring bowel gas anteriorly.

TRANSVERSE IMAGES

Transverse Plane/Anterior Approach

5. TRANSVERSE IMAGE OF THE DISTAL IVC TO INCLUDE THE HEPATIC VEINS.

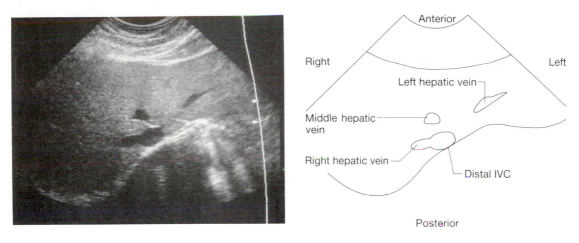

LABELED: IVC TRV DISTAL

6. TRANSVERSE IMAGE OF THE MIDDLE IVC AT THE LEVEL OF THE RENAL VEINS.

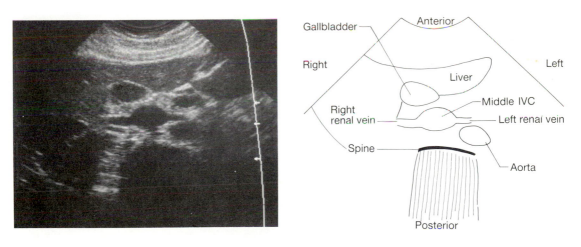

LABELED: IVC TRV MID

7. TRANSVERSE IMAGE OF THE PROXIMAL IVC.

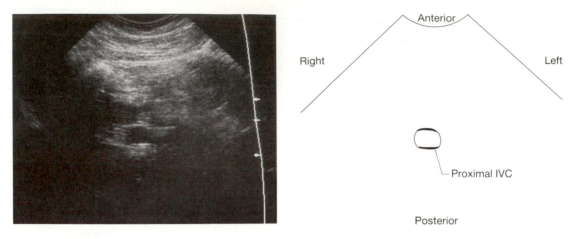

LABELED: IVC TRV PROX

8. TRANSVERSE IMAGE OF THE IVC BIFURCATION. (COMMON ILIAC VEINS).

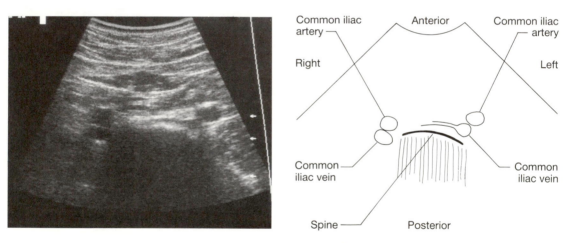

LABELED: IVC TRV BIF

NOTE: Measurements of the IVC are not required unless indicated by pathology.

REQUIRED PICTURES WHEN THE IVC IS NOT THE PRIMARY AREA OF INTEREST

1. LONGITUDINAL IMAGE OF THE DISTAL AND MIDDLE IVC.

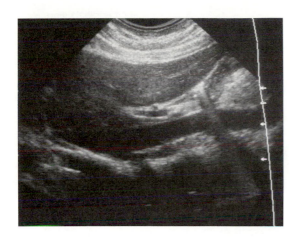
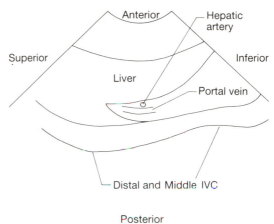

LABELED: IVC SAG DISTAL

2. TRANSVERSE IMAGE OF THE DISTAL IVC TO INCLUDE THE HEPATIC VEINS.

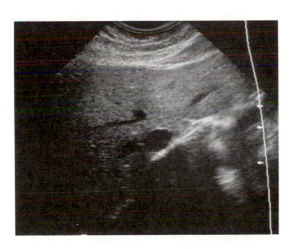
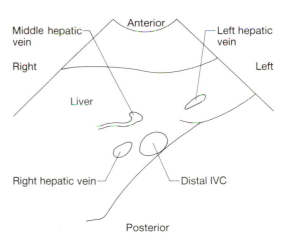

LABELED: IVC TRV DISTAL

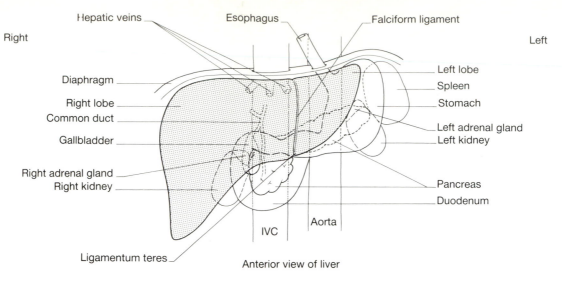

Anterior view of liver

Labels (clockwise from top): Hepatic veins, Esophagus, Falciform ligament, Right, Left, Diaphragm, Left lobe, Spleen, Right lobe, Stomach, Common duct, Left adrenal gland, Gallbladder, Left kidney, Right adrenal gland, Right kidney, Pancreas, Duodenum, Ligamentum teres, IVC, Aorta

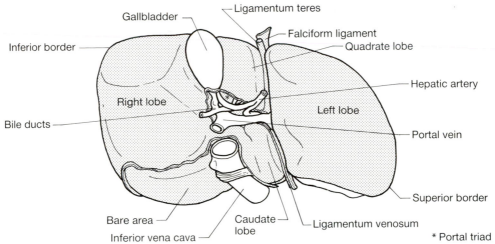

View of liver from below

Labels: Gallbladder, Ligamentum teres, Inferior border, Falciform ligament, Quadrate lobe, Hepatic artery, Right lobe, Left lobe, Bile ducts, Portal vein, Superior border, Bare area, Caudate lobe, Ligamentum venosum, Inferior vena cava, * Portal triad

Redrawn from Kapit W, Elson LM: The Anatomy Coloring Book. New York, Harper & Row, 1977.

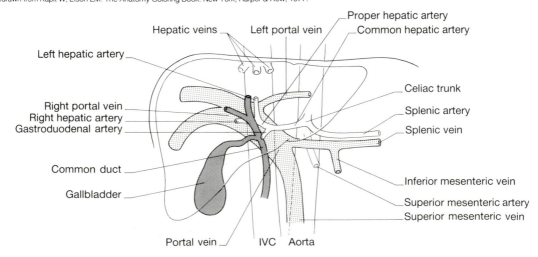

Vessels and ducts of liver

Labels: Hepatic veins, Left portal vein, Proper hepatic artery, Common hepatic artery, Left hepatic artery, Celiac trunk, Right portal vein, Splenic artery, Right hepatic artery, Splenic vein, Gastroduodenal artery, Common duct, Inferior mesenteric vein, Gallbladder, Superior mesenteric artery, Superior mesenteric vein, Portal vein, IVC, Aorta

ABDOMINAL ORGANS

CHAPTER SEVEN
LIVER SCANNING PROTOCOL

LOCATION

- Occupies the right upper quadrant and often extends past midline into the left upper quadrant.

- Intraperitoneal (except for a bare area that is posterior to the dome).

- Most anterior organ of the body.

- Superior and lateral surfaces border the diaphragm.

- The left lobe is just anterior to the stomach and body of the pancreas.

- The right lobe is just anterior to the gallbladder, right kidney (primarily superior pole), right adrenal gland, and head of the pancreas.

- The caudate lobe is posterior to the left lobe and anterior to the inferior vena cava.

ANATOMY

- Largest organ in the body.

- Size and shape are variable. Viewed anteriorly the liver has a basic wedge shape, tapering toward the left side. The right lobe is significantly larger than the left lobe.

- The hepatic artery, portal vein, and bile ducts pass through the porta hepatis or liver hilum.

- Lobes:
  - Right lobe.
  - Left lobe.
  - Caudate lobe.

NOTE: The medial portion of the left lobe is sometimes referred to as the quadrate lobe.

- Ligaments and main lobar fissure:
  - Main lobar fissure:
    Extends from the gallbladder to the right portal vein.
  - Ligamentum venosum:
    Separates caudate and left lobes.
  - Falciform ligament and ligamentum teres:
    Separates left lobe into medial and lateral portions.

49

- Vessels and ducts:
  - Hepatic veins:
    Carry the blood from the liver into the IVC.

  - Portal venous system:
    Carries the blood from the spleen and bowel to the liver. Portal vein formed by the confluence of the splenic vein, superior mesenteric vein, and inferior mesenteric vein.

  - Hepatic arteries:
    Carry oxygenated blood from the aorta to the liver.

  - Bile ducts:
    Carry bile, manufactured in the liver, to the duodenum.

  - Portal triad:
    Made up of the portal vein, hepatic artery, and bile duct.

PHYSIOLOGY

- Metabolism.
- Detoxifies drugs, toxins, and waste products of metabolism.
- Produces bile, needed for the digestion of fat.
- Stores glycogen, fats, copper, iron, and vitamins for physiological uses throughout the body.

SONOGRAPHIC APPEARANCE

- Lobes are midgray or medium-level echoes with even texture.

- Throughout, the lobes are portal and hepatic veins that are seen as branching, anechoic, tubular structures. To differentiate them, follow their branches back toward the porta hepatis or IVC, respectively.

NOTE: The major portal vein branches are surrounded by fibrofatty tissue and appear echogenic. Smaller portal vein branches may lack surrounding echoes. Echogenic walls can also be seen around the larger hepatic vein tributaries. Because of this variability, note that these features do not allow a reliable distinction between these two vessel systems.

- The only other normal structures that disrupt the otherwise uniform parenchymal liver texture are the echogenic ligaments and the structures at the porta hepatis: the portal triad (portal vein, hepatic artery, and bile duct), cystic duct, and neck of the gallbladder.

Normal Variants

- Reidel's lobe:
  Inferior extension of the right lobe.

- Absence of left lobe:
  Very rare. Results from occlusion of the left hepatic vein due to abnormal extension of neonatal spasm of the ligamentum venosum.

- Many variations in size and shape.

Patient Prep

- Fasting for 8 to 12 hours, because the gallbladder, biliary tract, and pancreas will be evaluated. This guarantees normal gallbladder and biliary tract dilatation and reduces the stomach and bowel gas anterior to the pancreas.

- If the patient has eaten, still do the liver exam.

NOTE: Liver evaluation is not usually limited by bowel gas, since the bowel tract is anatomically inferior to the liver.

Patient Position

- **Supine.**

- Left posterior oblique, left lateral decubitus, sitting semierect to erect or prone as needed.

NOTE: Different patient positions should be used whenever the suggested position does not give the desired results.

Transducer

- **3.0 MHz** or **3.5 MHz.**

- 5.0 MHz for very thin patient.

NOTE: It may be necessary to use 5.0 MHz for a patient's left lobe and 3.0 or 3.5 MHz on the right lobe.

Breathing Technique

- **Deep, held inspiration.**

NOTE: Different breathing techniques should be used whenever the suggested breathing technique does not give the desired results.

Liver Survey

LONGITUDINAL SURVEY

Sagittal Plane/Anterior Approach

• BEGIN WITH THE TRANSDUCER PER-PENDICULAR, AT THE MIDLINE OF THE BODY, JUST INFERIOR TO THE XIPHOID PROCESS OF THE STERNUM.

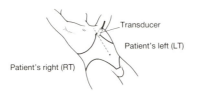

   THIS IS THE GENERAL AREA OF THE LEFT LOBE.
   NOTE THE LIGAMENTUM VENOSUM, CAUDATE LOBE, AND AORTA OR IVC.

NOTE: Depending on liver shape and patient respiration, varying degrees of subcostal and inferior angles may have to be used when scanning the liver longitudinally to completely survey the surperior and inferior liver margins. In some cases intercostal scanning will be necessary.

• WHILE VIEWING THE LEFT LOBE, USE SUBCOSTAL ANGLES AND MOVE THE TRANSDUCER TO THE PATIENT'S LEFT, LATERAL AND INFERIOR ALONG THE COSTAL MARGIN UNTIL YOU ARE BEYOND THE LEFT LOBE. NOTE THE AORTA.

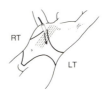

• RETURN TO MIDLINE, JUST INFERIOR TO THE XIPHOID PROCESS.

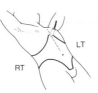

• TO EVALUATE THE RIGHT LOBE, USE SUBCOSTAL ANGLES AND MOVE THE TRANSDUCER TO THE PATIENT'S RIGHT, LATERAL AND INFERIOR ALONG THE COSTAL MARGIN UNTIL YOU ARE BEYOND THE RIGHT LATERAL, INFERIOR LOBE.

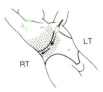

NOTE THE IVC, HEPATIC VEINS, POR-
TAL VEIN, PORTAL TRIAD, PORTA HEPA-
TIS, MAIN LOBAR FISSURE, BILE DUCTS,
GALLBLADDER, RIGHT KIDNEY, AND PERI-
NEPHRIC SPACE.

● MOVE THE TRANSDUCER BACK ONTO
THE RIGHT LATERAL INFERIOR LOBE.
PLACE THE TRANSDUCER AT THE MOST
LATERAL EDGE OF THE RIGHT COSTAL
MARGIN AND USE A VERY SHARP SUB-
COSTAL ANGLE TO VIEW THE RIGHT LAT-
ERAL SUPERIOR LOBE. MOVE OR ANGLE
THE TRANSDUCER RIGHT LATERAL AND
SWEEP THROUGH AND BEYOND THE
RIGHT LATERAL SUPERIOR LOBE.

NOTE THE DOME OF THE RIGHT LOBE
AND ADJACENT PLEURAL SPACE.

N O T E : The longitudinal of the right lateral superior lobe can be difficult to visualize from a sagittal plane subcostal angle.
Sagittal plane intercostal scanning or
right coronal plane subcostal or intercostal scanning can be used.

Sagittal Plane/Anterior Intercostal Approach

● **Patient supine,** left posterior oblique or
sitting semierect to erect.

● Begin with the transducer perpendicular in an intercostal space immediately
anterior to the right lateral superior
lobe.

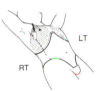

● Suspended respiration should make the
area more viewable.

● Move the transducer to adjacent intercostal spaces to evaluate the entire right
lateral superior lobe.

● Angling the transducer within the intercostal spaces and using different breathing techniques can aid evaluation.

● Note the dome of the right lobe and adjacent pleural space.

*Coronal Plane/Right Lateral Subcostal
Approach*

- Patient **supine**, left posterior oblique,
  left lateral decubitus, sitting semierect
  to erect.

- Begin with the transducer angled sub-
  costally, midcoronal plane. Varying degrees of subcostal angles and deep, held
  respiration should make the right lateral superior lobe viewable.

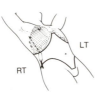

- Note the dome of the right lobe and adjacent pleural space.

*Coronal Plane/Right Lateral Intercostal
Approach*

- Patient **supine**, left posterior oblique,
  left lateral decubitus, sitting semierect
  to erect.

- Begin with the transducer perpendicular, midcoronal plane, just inferior to
  the costal margin. Move superiorly into
  the first intercostal space.

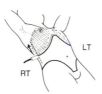

- Using suspended or deep, held respiration, move superiorly through the adjacent intercostal spaces until you scan
  through and beyond the right lateral superior lobe.

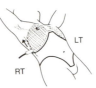

- Angling the transducer within the intercostal spaces and using different breathing techniques can aid evaluation.

- Note the dome of the right lobe and adjacent pleural space.

TRANSVERSE SURVEY

Transverse Plane/Anterior Approach

● BEGIN WITH THE TRANSDUCER PER-PENDICULAR, AT THE MIDLINE OF THE BODY, JUST INFERIOR TO THE XIPHOID PROCESS OF THE STERNUM.

THIS IS THE GENERAL AREA OF THE LEFT LOBE.

NOTE THE LIGAMENTUM VENOSUM, CAUDATE LOBE, HEPATIC VEIN(S), IVC, AND AORTA.

NOTE: Depending on liver shape and patient respiration, varying degrees of subcostal and inferior angles may have to be used when scanning the liver transversely to completely survey the superior and inferior liver margins. In some cases intercostal scanning may be necessary.

● WHILE VIEWING THE LEFT LOBE, MOVE THE TRANSDUCER INFERIOR UNTIL YOU SCAN THROUGH AND BEYOND THE LEFT LOBE. NOTE THE PORTAL VEIN AND LIG-AMENTUM TERES.

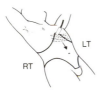

● DEPENDING ON LIVER SHAPE AND SIZE, ALL OF THE LEFT LATERAL ASPECT OF THE LEFT LOBE MAY BE SEEN IN ITS EN-TIRETY FROM MIDLINE. IF NOT, RETURN TO MIDLINE, JUST INFERIOR TO THE XI-PHOID PROCESS. USE SUBCOSTAL AND INFERIOR ANGLES AND MOVE THE TRANSDUCER TO THE PATIENT'S LEFT, LATERAL AND INFERIOR ALONG THE COS-TAL MARGIN UNTIL YOU ARE BEYOND THE LEFT LOBE.

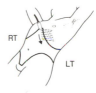

● RETURN TO MIDLINE, JUST INFERIOR TO THE XIPHOID PROCESS.

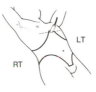

● TO EVALUATE THE RIGHT LOBE, USE SUBCOSTAL AND INFERIOR ANGLES AND MOVE THE TRANSDUCER TO THE PATIENT'S RIGHT, LATERAL AND INFERIOR ALONG THE COSTAL MARGIN UNTIL YOU ARE BEYOND THE RIGHT LATERAL INFERIOR LOBE.

NOTE THE IVC, HEPATIC VEINS, PORTAL VEIN, PORTAL TRIAD, RIGHT AND LEFT PORTAL BRANCHES, PORTA HEPATIS, MAIN LOBAR FISSURE, BILE DUCTS, GALLBLADDER, RIGHT KIDNEY, AND PERINEPHRIC SPACE.

● MOVE THE TRANSDUCER BACK ONTO THE RIGHT LATERAL INFERIOR LOBE. PLACE THE TRANSDUCER AT THE MOST LATERAL EDGE OF THE RIGHT COSTAL MARGIN AND USE A VERY SHARP SUBCOSTAL ANGLE TO VIEW THE RIGHT LATERAL SUPERIOR LOBE. MOVE OR ANGLE THE TRANSDUCER RIGHT LATERAL AND SWEEP THROUGH AND BEYOND THE RIGHT LATERAL SUPERIOR LOBE. NOTE THE DOME OF THE RIGHT LOBE AND ADJACENT PLEURAL SPACE.

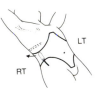

NOTE: The transverse of the right lateral superior lobe can be difficult to visualize from a transverse plane subcostal angle. Transverse plane intercostal scanning or transverse plane right lateral subcostal or right lateral intercostal scanning can be used.

Transverse plane/anterior intercostal approach

Transverse plane/right lateral subcostal approach

Transverse plane/right lateral intercostal approach

Use the same suggested scanning methods as those for the longitudinal surveys of the right lateral superior lobe.

REQUIRED PICTURES

LONGITUDINAL IMAGES

Sagittal Plane/Anterior Approach

1. LONGITUDINAL IMAGE OF THE LEFT LOBE TO INCLUDE THE INFERIOR MARGIN AND THE AORTA.

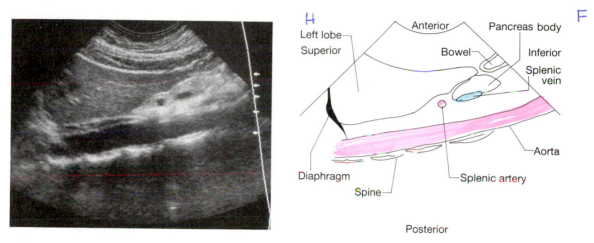

LABELED: LIVER SAG LT LOBE

2. LONGITUDINAL IMAGE OF THE LEFT LOBE TO INCLUDE THE DIAPHRAGM AND CAUDATE LOBE.

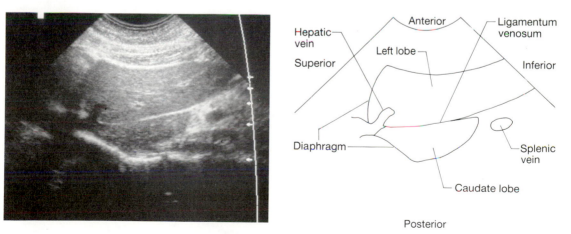

LABELED: LIVER SAG LT LOBE

3. LONGITUDINAL IMAGE OF THE RIGHT LOBE TO INCLUDE THE IVC WHERE IT PASSES THROUGH THE LIVER.

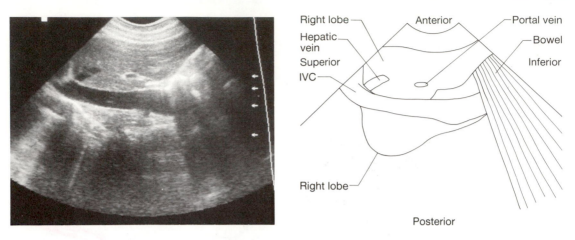

LABELED: LIVER SAG RT LOBE

4. LONGITUDINAL IMAGE OF THE RIGHT LOBE TO INCLUDE THE MAIN LOBAR FISSURE, GALLBLADDER, AND PORTAL VEIN.

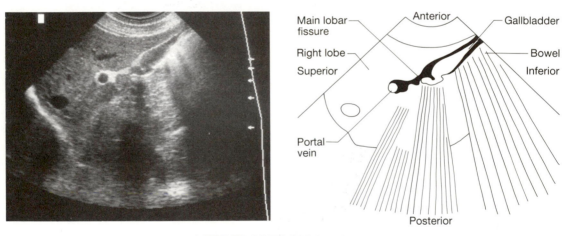

LABELED: LIVER SAG RT LOBE

5. LONGITUDINAL IMAGE OF THE RIGHT LOBE TO INCLUDE PART OF THE RIGHT KIDNEY FOR PARENCHYMA COMPARISON.

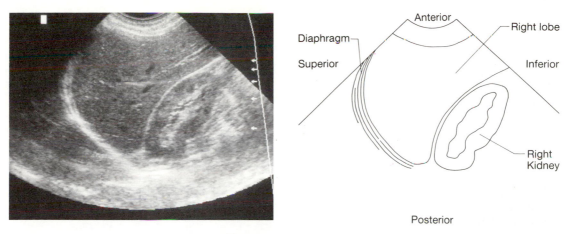

LABELED: LIVER SAG RT LOBE

6. LONGITUDINAL IMAGE OF THE RIGHT LOBE TO INCLUDE THE DOME AND THE ADJACENT PLEURAL SPACE.

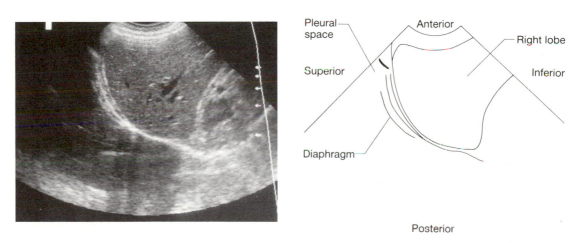

LABELED: LIVER SAG RT LOBE

TRANSVERSE IMAGES

Transverse Plane/Anterior Approach

7. TRANSVERSE IMAGE OF THE LEFT LOBE TO INCLUDE ITS LATERAL MARGIN.

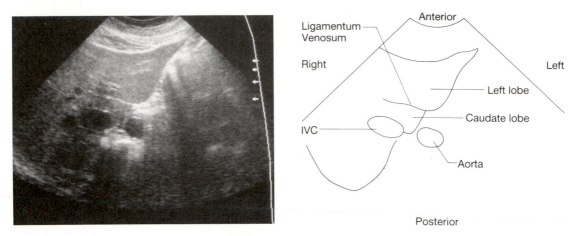

LABELED: LIVER TRV LT LOBE

8. TRANSVERSE IMAGE OF THE LEFT LOBE TO INCLUDE THE LIGAMENTUM TERES.

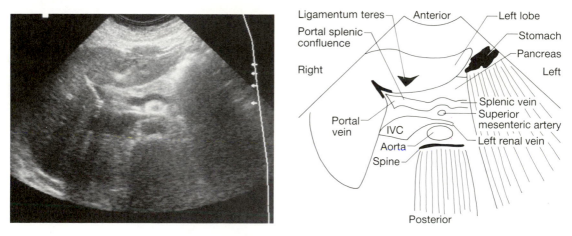

LABELED: LIVER TRV LT LOBE

NOTE: Depending on liver size and shape it may be possible to take a transverse image that includes the left lobe's lateral margin and the ligamentum teres. If so, label: liver trv. lt. lobe

9. TRANSVERSE IMAGE OF THE RIGHT LOBE TO INCLUDE THE HEPATIC VEINS.

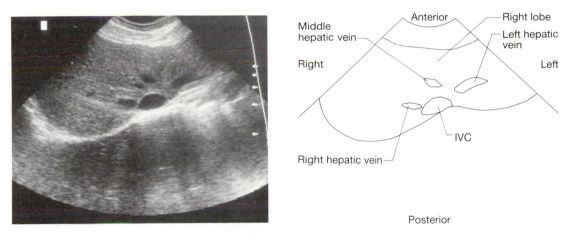

LABELED: LIVER TRV RT LOBE

10. TRANSVERSE IMAGE OF THE RIGHT LOBE TO INCLUDE THE RIGHT AND LEFT BRANCHES OF THE PORTAL VEIN.

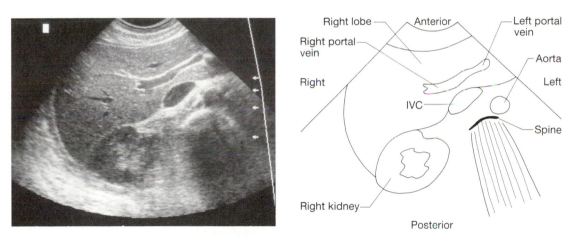

LABELED: LIVER TRV RT LOBE

11. TRANSVERSE IMAGE OF THE RIGHT LATERAL INFERIOR LOBE.

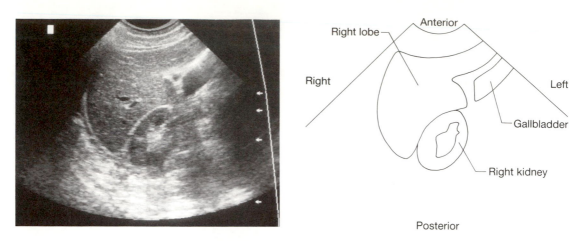

LABELED: LIVER TRV RT LOBE

12. TRANSVERSE IMAGE OF THE RIGHT LOBE TO INCLUDE THE DOME AND THE ADJACENT PLEURAL SPACE.

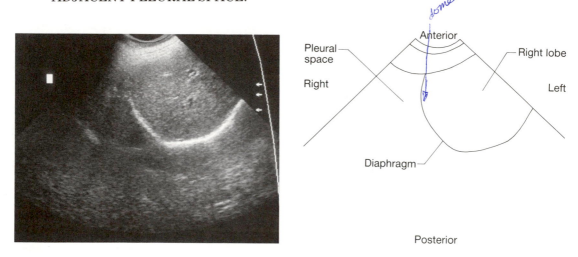

LABELED: LIVER TRV RT LOBE

NOTE: Measurements of the liver are not required unless indicated by pathology.

REQUIRED PICTURES WHEN THE LIVER IS NOT THE PRIMARY AREA OF INTEREST

REQUIRED PICTURES ARE THE SAME AS THOSE REQUIRED FOR THE LIVER SURVEY.

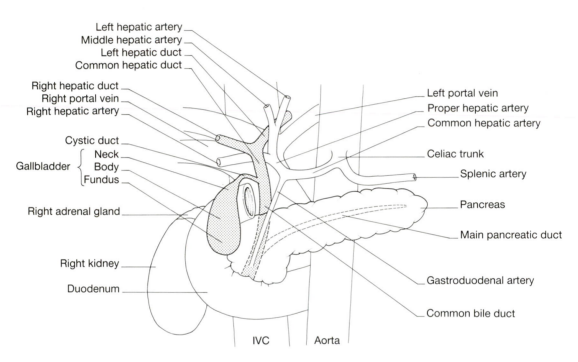

Location and anatomy of the gallbladder and biliary tract

Left hepatic artery
Middle hepatic artery
Left hepatic duct
Common hepatic duct

Right hepatic duct
Right portal vein
Right hepatic artery

Cystic duct

Gallbladder { Neck
Body
Fundus

Right adrenal gland

Right kidney

Duodenum

Left portal vein
Proper hepatic artery
Common hepatic artery

Celiac trunk

Splenic artery

Pancreas

Main pancreatic duct

Gastroduodenal artery

Common bile duct

IVC   Aorta

CHAPTER EIGHT
GALLBLADDER AND BILIARY TRACT SCANNING PROTOCOL

LOCATION

- Right upper quadrant.

- Intraperitoneal.

- Immediately posterior to the liver.

- Neck of the gallbladder is fixed in its position at the main lobar fissure.

- Body and fundus of the gallbladder are extremely variable in position.

- Fundus of the gallbladder may be anterior to the superior pole of the right kidney.

- Cystic duct is superior to the gallbladder neck.

- Common bile duct is inferior to the gallbladder. It can also be posterior to the gallbladder, depending on the lie of the gallbladder.

- Common bile duct is right lateral to the common hepatic artery.

- Common duct is anterior to the portal vein.

ANATOMY

- Right and left hepatic ducts exit from the liver at the porta hepatis and meet to form the common duct.

- The superior (proximal) portion of the common duct is referred to as the common hepatic duct, and the inferior (distal) portion as the common bile duct.

- The common hepatic duct courses inferomedially and meets with the cystic duct of the gallbladder to form the common bile duct.

- The common bile duct courses inferomedially running behind the duodenum on its way to the head of the pancreas.

- The common bile duct either passes through the pancreatic head or runs along a groove on its posterior surface to meet with the main pancreatic duct. Joined together or separately, the ducts enter the duodenum at the ampulla of Vater.

- The gallbladder is pear-shaped. Its rounded inferior portion is the fundus and its superior tapering portion is the neck. The middle portion of the gallbladder is referred to as its body.

- Normal gallbladder size is variable according to the amount of bile it is storing. Up to 3 cm wide and 7 cm to 10 cm long is normal size for the gallbladder.

- Normal common duct size is variable according to the amount of bile in it and patient age. Common duct may enlarge with age.

- Up to 4 mm is normal for the common hepatic duct near the porta hepatis.

- Up to 7 mm is normal for the common bile duct distally.

NOTE: The common duct assumes bile storage function following loss of gallbladder function resulting from cholecystectomy or gallbladder disease. Up to 10 mm is normal for size.

- The cystic duct connects the gallbladder neck with the common duct.

- The area where the cystic duct and gallbladder neck join is tortuous and referred to as the spiral valve. This reference is to appearance only because there is no valvular action.

PHYSIOLOGY

- Accessory to the digestive system.

- Liver manufactures bile, a fat emulsifier and carrier of liver waste. Bile is stored and concentrated in the gallbladder, then travels via the bile ducts to the small intestine when needed to aid digestion.

SONOGRAPHIC APPEARANCE

- The bile-filled gallbladder is an anechoic oblong structure with echogenic walls.

- The bile-filled common duct is an anechoic tubular structure with echogenic walls.

NORMAL VARIANTS

- Shape variations:
  - Segmental contractions that disappear after fasting or changing patient position.
  - Phrygian cap is an example of where the gallbladder fundus is folded over.

- Position variations:
  - The gallbladder can be found throughout the abdomen because it is suspended on long mesentery.
  - Very rare deep fossa intrahepatic gallbladder.

- Septations:
  - May partially or totally divide the gallbladder.
  - May partially or totally divide the cystic duct, producing various degrees of double gallbladder.

- Duplication of the common duct:
  - Very rare. Can be partial or complete.

- The level of the junction of the cystic duct and common hepatic duct is variable.

PATIENT PREP

- Fasting for 8 to 12 hours to guarantee maximum gallbladder and biliary tract dilatation but may be scanned after 4 to 6 hours.

NOTE: Before a gallbladder exam it is very important to determine when a patient last ate because the inability to visualize the gallbladder with ultrasound is indicative of gallbladder disease.

PATIENT POSITION

- **Supine** and **left lateral decubitus.**
- Left posterior oblique, sitting semierect to erect or prone as needed.

NOTE: Biliary system examinations must be done in two patient positions. This allows for differentiation between pathologies. For example, gallstones and sludge move, and other considerations such as polyps and gallbladder carcinoma are stationary.

NOTE: Different patient positions should be used whenever the suggested position does not give the desired results.

TRANSDUCER

- **3.0 MHz** or **3.5 MHz.**
- 5.0 MHz for thin patients and anterior-lying gallbladders.

BREATHING TECHNIQUE

- **Deep, held inspiration.**

NOTE: Different breathing techniques should be used whenever the suggested breathing technique does not give the desired results.

GALLBLADDER SURVEY

NOTE: Gallbladder and biliary tract surveys **must be done in two patient positions.** Use the following scanning methods for both positions.

LONGITUDINAL SURVEY

Sagittal Plane/Anterior Approach

● BEGIN WITH THE TRANSDUCER PERPENDICULAR, JUST INFERIOR TO THE COSTAL MARGIN AT THE RIGHT MEDIAL ANGLE OF THE RIBS.

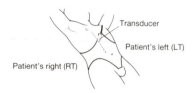

USUALLY THIS IS THE AREA OF THE PORTAL VEIN AND GALLBLADDER NECK. IF THE GALLBLADDER IS NOT SEEN HERE, FIND THE MAIN LOBAR FISSURE THAT EXTENDS FROM THE GALLBLADDER TO THE RIGHT PORTAL VEIN.

NOTE: Subcostal transducer angles can help locate the gallbladder. In some cases intercostal scanning will be necessary. Also, the gallbladder tends to lie in the area between the right medial angle of the ribs and the superior pole of the right kidney Therefore, moving the transducer inferior and right lateral can be another way to locate the gallbladder.

● ONCE THE GALLBLADDER IS LOCATED, DETERMINE ITS LONGITUDINAL LIE. THIS CAN BE ACCOMPLISHED BY ROTATING THE TRANSDUCER TO OBLIQUE THE SCANNING PLANE. OCCASIONALLY, NO OBLIQUE IS REQUIRED.

NOTE: The longitudinal of the gallbladder can lie in either the sagittal plane or transverse plane because of the variability in gallbladder position.

● ASSUMING THE LONGITUDINAL IS SEEN IN AN OBLIQUE SAGITTAL PLANE, SLIGHTLY ROCK THE TRANSDUCER RIGHT TO LEFT, SWEEPING THROUGH BOTH SIDES OF THE GALLBLADDER, AND AT THE SAME TIME SLIDE INFERIORLY THROUGH AND BEYOND THE FUNDUS.

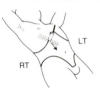

● ROCKING AND SLIDING, MOVE THE TRANSDUCER SUPERIORLY BACK ONTO THE FUNDUS AND CONTINUE SCANNING UP THROUGH THE BODY AND NECK UNTIL YOU ARE BEYOND THE GALLBLADDER.

TRANSVERSE SURVEY

Transverse Plane/Anterior Approach

● STILL IN THE SAGITTAL SCANNING PLANE, LOCATE THE FUNDUS OF THE GALLBLADDER. ROTATE THE TRANSDUCER 90 DEGREES INTO THE TRANSVERSE SCANNING PLANE AND TRAVERSE THE FUNDUS. THE FUNDUS WILL APPEAR ROUND OR OVAL.

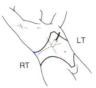

NOTE: An optional method for locating the gallbladder in the transverse plane is locating the superior pole of the right kidney first. In most cases, the fundus of the gallbladder is seen immediately anterior to the superior right pole.

● SLIGHTLY ROCK THE TRANSDUCER SUPERIOR TO INFERIOR AND AT THE SAME TIME SLIDE INFERIORLY THROUGH AND BEYOND THE FUNDUS.

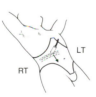

● CONTINUE ROCKING AND SLIDE THE TRANSDUCER SUPERIORLY BACK ONTO THE FUNDUS AND CONTINUE SCANNING UP THROUGH THE BODY AND NECK UNTIL YOU ARE BEYOND THE GALLBLADDER.

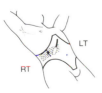

BILIARY TRACT SURVEY

LONGITUDINAL SURVEY

Sagittal Plane/Anterior Approach

● BEGIN BY LOCATING THE NECK OF THE GALLBLADDER OR THE MAIN LOBAR FISSURE. NOTE THE PORTAL VEIN AND LOOK FOR THE LONGITUDINAL OF THE COMMON DUCT ANTERIORLY. IT MAY BE NECESSARY TO ROTATE THE TRANSDUCER AT VARYING DEGREES (TO OBLIQUE THE SCANNING PLANE ACCORDING TO THE LIE OF THE DUCT) TO VISUALIZE THE LONG AXIS OF THE COMMON DUCT. NOTE THAT THE COMMON DUCT USUALLY LIES AT A RIGHT ANGLE TO THE COSTAL MARGIN.

NOTE: In a sagittal oblique plane the portal vein at the level of the porta hepatis will be traversed, seen as round or oval. Inferior to this the portal vein appears longitudinal as it runs posterior and parallel to the duct.

● *SLIGHTLY* ROCK THE TRANSDUCER RIGHT TO LEFT SWEEPING THROUGH BOTH SIDES OF THE DUCT AND AT THE SAME TIME *SLOWLY* SLIDE THE TRANSDUCER *SLIGHTLY* SUPERIOR AND RIGHT LATERAL THROUGH AND BEYOND THE COMMON HEPATIC DUCT.

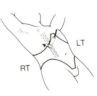

NOTE THAT THE DISTANCE YOU MOVE IS SMALL.

NOTE THE TRAVERSED HEPATIC ARTERY BETWEEN THE DUCT AND THE PORTAL VEIN.

• MOVE THE TRANSDUCER BACK ONTO THE COMMON HEPATIC DUCT AND RETURN TO THE LEVEL OF THE GALLBLADDER NECK OR MAIN LOBAR FISSURE.

• CONTINUE BY *SLIGHTLY* ROCKING THE TRANSDUCER RIGHT TO LEFT AND AT THE SAME TIME *SLOWLY* SLIDE THE TRANSDUCER *SLIGHTLY* INFERIOR AND MEDIAL THROUGH THE COMMON BILE DUCT TO THE HEAD OF THE PANCREAS.

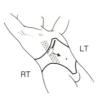

NOTE THAT THE DISTANCE YOU MOVE IS SMALL.

NOTE THE TRAVERSED HEPATIC ARTERY BETWEEN THE DUCT AND THE PORTAL VEIN.

STAY AT THIS LOCATION TO BEGIN THE TRANSVERSE SURVEY.

NOTE: The common bile duct can be difficult to see when it is behind the duodenum because of bowel gas. Continue to scan through the duodenum and pick up the duct again just inferior to the duodenum or at the head of the pancreas. Giving the patient enough water to drink to fill the duodenum can aid in the evaluation of the retroduodenal portion of the common bile duct, as the water displaces the bowel gas.

TRANSVERSE SURVEY

Transverse Plane/Anterior Approach

NOTE: Because of the small size of the common duct, transverse evaluation can be difficult. Therefore, common hepatic duct (proximal) evaluation is done at the gallbladder neck and common bile duct (distal) evaluation is done at the head of the pancreas.

• STILL IN THE SAGITTAL SCANNING PLANE EVALUATING THE LONGITUDINAL OF THE COMMON BILE DUCT AT THE HEAD OF THE PANCREAS, ROTATE THE TRANSDUCER 90 DEGREES INTO THE TRANSVERSE SCANNING PLANE AND TRAVERSE THE COMMON BILE DUCT.

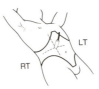

• IF YOU LOSE SIGHT OF THE DUCT WHILE ROTATING THE TRANSDUCER, LOOK FOR THE SMALL, ROUND OR OVAL DUCT IN THE LATERAL AND POSTERIOR PORTIONS OF THE PANCREATIC HEAD. NOTE THE TRAVERSED GASTRODUODENAL ARTERY ANTERIOR TO THE DUCT.

• RETURN TO THE SAGITTAL SCANNING PLANE AND LOCATE THE NECK OF THE GALLBLADDER AND JUST SUPERIOR TO IT THE LONGITUDINAL COMMON HEPATIC DUCT. ROTATE THE TRANSDUCER 90 DEGREES INTO THE TRANSVERSE SCANNING PLANE AND TRAVERSE THE COMMON HEPATIC DUCT.

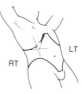

• IF YOU LOSE SIGHT OF THE DUCT WHILE ROTATING THE TRANSDUCER, LOOK FOR THE SMALL, ROUND OR OVAL DUCT ANTERIOR TO THE PORTAL VEIN.

REQUIRED PICTURES

NOTE: Gallbladder and biliary tract pictures **must be done in two patient positions.**

FIRST POSITION/SUPINE

Longitudinal Gallbladder Images
Sagittal Plane/Anterior Approach

1. LONG AXIS IMAGE OF THE GALLBLADDER.

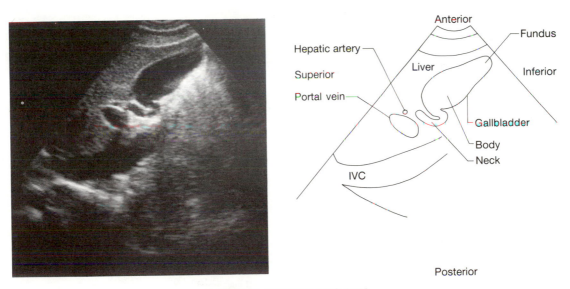

LABELED: GB SAG LONG AXIS

NOTE: In many cases gallbladder definition is sacrificed to achieve the long axis. Therefore, additional longitudinal images of the gallbladder fundus, body, and neck should be taken.

2. LONGITUDINAL IMAGE OF THE GALLBLADDER FUNDUS AND BODY.

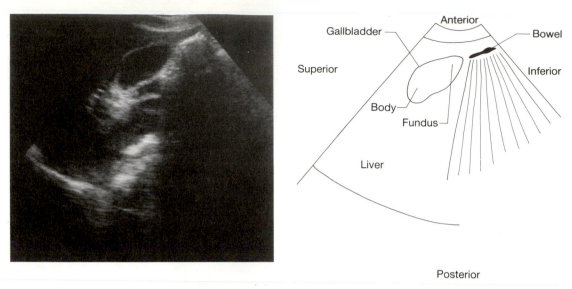

LABELED: GB SAG FUNDUS/BODY

3. LONGITUDINAL IMAGE OF THE GALLBLADDER NECK.

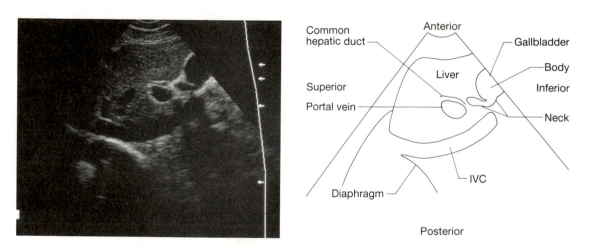

LABELED: GB SAG NECK

Transverse Gallbladder Images

Transverse Plane/Anterior Approach

4. TRANSVERSE IMAGE OF THE GALLBLADDER FUNDUS.

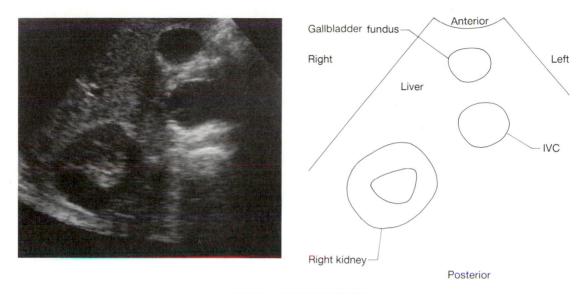

LABELED: GB TRV FUNDUS

5. TRANSVERSE IMAGE OF THE GALLBLADDER BODY.

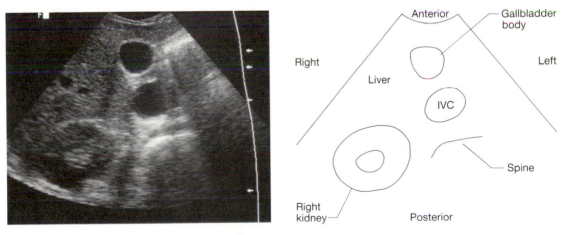

LABELED: GB TRV BODY

6. TRANSVERSE IMAGE OF THE GALLBLADDER NECK.

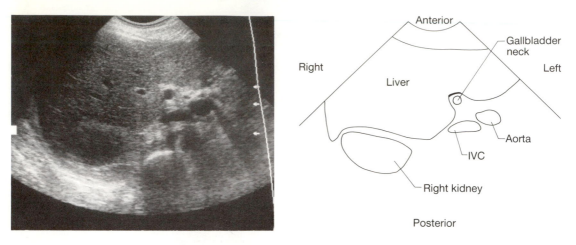

LABELED: GB TRV NECK

Longitudinal Biliary Tract Images

Sagittal Plane/Anterior Approach

NOTE: Images of the common duct may be taken in the second patient position if they were better visualized there during the survey.

NOTE: Images of the common duct can be magnified to aid interpretation.

7. LONGITUDINAL IMAGE OF THE COMMON HEPATIC DUCT.

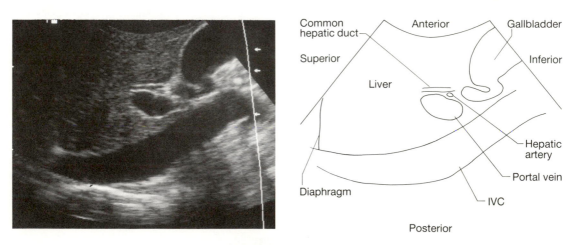

LABELED: SAG CHD

NOTE: The longitudinal common hepatic duct image can be eliminated if the common hepatic duct was imaged with the gallbladder long axis image or longitudinal neck image.

8. LONGITUDINAL IMAGE OF THE COMMON BILE DUCT WITH *ANTERIOR TO POSTERIOR MEASUREMENT*.

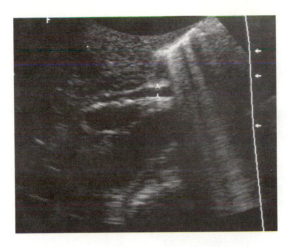

LABELED: SAG CBD

9. SAME IMAGE AS NUMBER 8 WITHOUT CALIPERS.

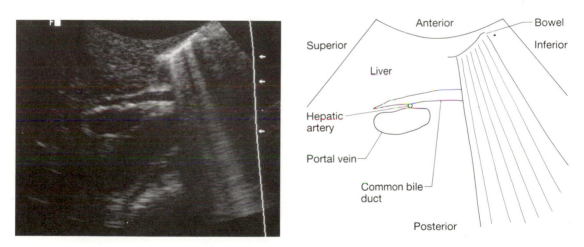

LABELED: SAG CBD

NOTE: Measurement of the duct should be at the widest part of the lumen.

SECOND POSITION/LEFT LATERAL DECUBITUS

Longitudinal Gallbladder Image

Sagittal Plane/Anterior Approach

1. LONG AXIS IMAGE OF THE GALLBLADDER.

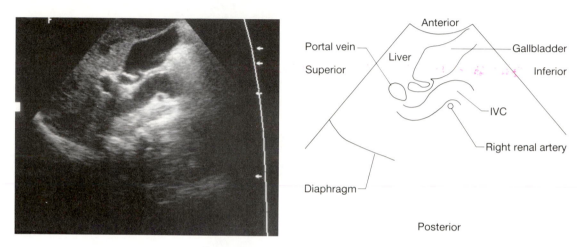

LABELED: GB SAG LONG AXIS

Transverse Gallbladder Image

Transverse Plane/Anterior Approach

2. TRANSVERSE IMAGE OF THE GALLBLADDER FUNDUS.

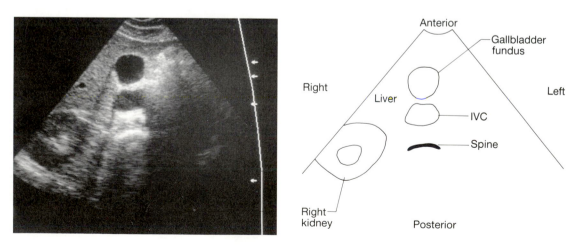

LABELED: GB TRV FUNDUS

REQUIRED PICTURES WHEN THE GALLBLADDER AND BILIARY TRACT ARE NOT THE PRIMARY AREA OF INTEREST

SINGLE POSITION

Longitudinal Gallbladder Image

Sagittal Plane/Anterior Approach

1. LONG AXIS IMAGE OF THE GALLBLADDER.

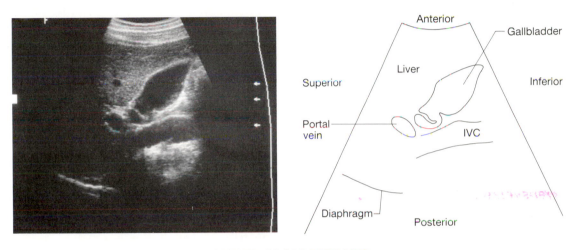

LABELED: GB SAG LONG AXIS

Transverse Gallbladder Image

Transverse Plane/Anterior Approach

2. TRANSVERSE IMAGE OF THE GALLBLADDER FUNDUS.

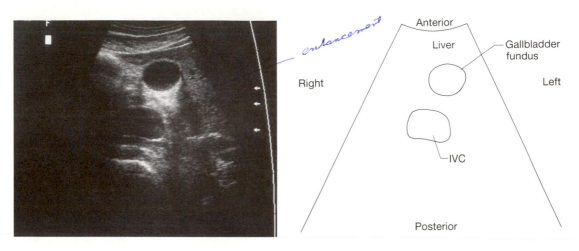

LABELED: GB TRV FUNDUS

Longitudinal Biliary Tract Images

Sagittal Plane/Anterior Approach

NOTE: Images of the common duct can be magnified to aid interpretation.

3. LONGITUDINAL IMAGE OF THE COMMON HEPATIC DUCT.

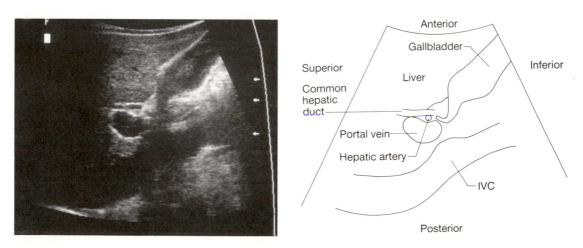

LABELED: SAG CHD

NOTE: The longitudinal common hepatic duct image can be eliminated if the common hepatic duct was imaged with the gallbladder long axis image.

4. LONGITUDINAL IMAGE OF THE COMMON BILE DUCT WITH *ANTERIOR TO POSTERIOR MEASUREMENT*.

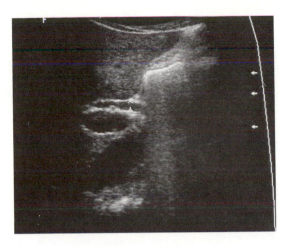

LABELED: SAG CBD

5. SAME IMAGE AS NUMBER 4 WITHOUT CALIPERS.

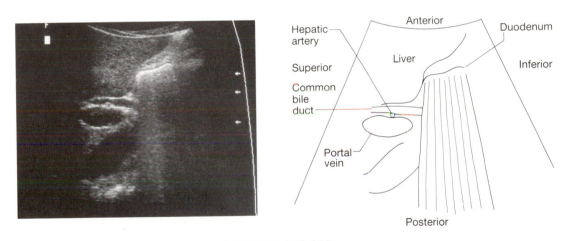

LABELED: SAG CBD

NOTE: Measurement of the duct should be at the widest part of the lumen.

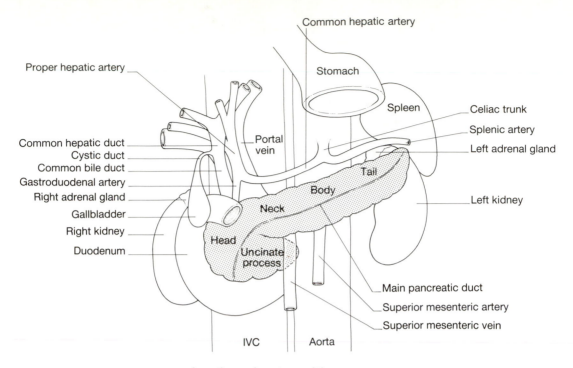

Location and anatomy of the pancreas

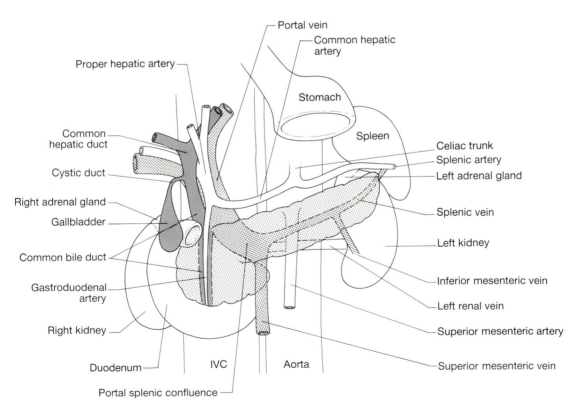

Location and anatomy of the pancreas

CHAPTER NINE
PANCREAS SCANNING PROTOCOL

LOCATION

- Traverses the body, extending from the hilum of the spleen to the duodenum.

- Retroperitoneal.

- Pancreas head and uncinate are anterior to the IVC.

- The uncinate is posterior to the superior mesenteric vein.

- Pancreas neck is anterior to the superior mesenteric vein.

- Pancreas body is posterior to the stomach.

- Pancreas body is anterior to the splenic vein, superior mesenteric artery, right renal vein, and aorta.

- Pancreas body and tail are inferior to the splenic artery.

- Pancreas tail is anterior to the splenic vein and left kidney.

ANATOMY

- The pancreas is 15 to 20 cm long, and though it is not actually segmented, it is described in segments:

  - Head:
    Lies to the right of the superior mesenteric vein against the medial curve of the duodenum and immediately anterior to the IVC.
    The gastroduodenal artery lies at the anterolateral border. The common bile duct lies at the posterolateral border.
    The anterior to posterior dimensions of the head range from 2.0 to 2.5 cm.

  - Uncinate process:
    The medial portion of the head that lies immediately posterior to the superior mesenteric vein. Variable in size, it can extend left lateral and lie immediately posterior to the superior mesenteric artery.

  - Neck:
    Lies immediately anterior to the superior mesenteric vein, and slightly superior to that level lies anterior to the formation of the portal vein.
    The anterior to posterior dimensions of the neck range from 1.0 to 2.0 cm.

– Body:
Lies to the left of the neck, immediately anterior to the splenic vein, and extends left lateral toward the pancreas tail.
The anterior to posterior dimensions of the body range from 1.0 to 2.0 cm.

– Tail:
Lies to the left of the pancreas body, immediately anterior to the splenic vein, and extends left lateral to the hilum of the spleen.
The anterior to posterior dimensions of the tail range from 1.0 to 2.0 cm.

- Size, shape, and lie are variable. Viewed anteriorly the pancreas can be seen head to tail, with the head appearing slightly larger.

- The pancreas decreases in size with age.

- Wirsung's duct, the main pancreatic duct, extends the length of the pancreas and enlarges toward the head up to 3 mm. It meets with the common bile duct at the pancreas head, and joined together or separately the ducts enter the duodenum.

- Santorini's duct, an accessory duct, is small and sometimes absent. It enters the duodenum separately from Wirsung's duct.

PHYSIOLOGY

- Endocrine function produces the hormone insulin to prevent diabetes mellitus.

- Exocrine function produces pancreatic enzymes that, via the pancreatic duct(s), aid digestion.

SONOGRAPHIC APPEARANCE

- Pancreas is midgray or medium-level echoes with even texture that is equal to or more echogenic than the normal liver.

- The pancreas becomes more echogenic with age.

- The contour of the normal pancreas should always be smooth.

NOTE: The pancreas is not encapsulated, and therefore retroperitoneal fat may infiltrate the gland and make the contour difficult to evaluate.

- Wirsung's duct and Santorini's duct are anechoic tubular structures with echogenic walls.

NORMAL VARIANTS

- Size, shape, and lie are variable.

PATIENT PREP

- Fasting for 8 to 12 hours to reduce the stomach and bowel gas anterior to the pancreas. Also to ensure gallbladder and biliary tract dilatation for evaluation because certain pathologies of the pancreas, gallbladder, and biliary tract affect each other.

- If the patient has eaten, still do the exam. Stomach content can displace gas and act as a window for the sound beam. For this reason, 2 to 4 cups of water or noncarbonated drink can be given to the patient to aid evaluation if gas is obscuring the pancreas. This fluid technique works best if the patient is sitting erect.

- Peristalsis can cause the fluid to pass quickly through the stomach and duodenum, making evaluation of the pancreas inadequate. Peristaltic reducing drugs such as glucagon can be given to prevent this.

PATIENT POSITION

- **Supine.**

- Sitting semierect to erect, left posterior oblique, left lateral decubitus, or prone as needed.

NOTE: Different patient positions should be used whenever the suggested position does not give the desired results.

TRANSDUCER

- **3.0 MHz** or **3.5 MHz.**

- 5.0 MHz for thin patients and the anterior lying pancreas.

BREATHING TECHNIQUE

- **Deep, held inspiration.**

NOTE: Different breathing techniques should be used whenever the suggested breathing technique does not give the desired results.

PANCREAS SURVEY

NOTE: While surveying the pancreas, evaluate the peripancreatic regions for adenopathy.

LONGITUDINAL SURVEY

Transverse Plane/Anterior Approach

- BEGIN WITH THE TRANSDUCER PERPENDICULAR, AT THE MIDLINE OF THE BODY, JUST INFERIOR TO THE XIPHOID PROCESS OF THE STERNUM.

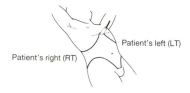

Patient's left (LT)
Patient's right (RT)

- SLIGHTLY ROCK THE TRANSDUCER SUPERIOR TO INFERIOR AND SLOWLY SLIDE THE TRANSDUCER INFERIORLY.

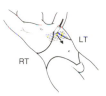

LT
RT

NOTE THAT THE BODY OF THE PANCREAS LIES JUST INFERIOR TO THE TRAVERSED CELIAC TRUNK AND LONGITUDINAL SPLENIC ARTERY AND JUST ANTERIOR TO THE LONGITUDINAL SPLENIC VEIN, WHICH IS IMMEDIATELY ANTERIOR TO THE TRAVERSED SUPERIOR MESENTERIC ARTERY.

- ONCE YOU LOCATE THE PANCREAS BODY, IT MAY BE NECESSARY TO ROTATE THE TRANSDUCER AT VARYING DEGREES (TO OBLIQUE THE SCANNING PLANE ACCORDING TO THE LIE OF THE PANCREAS) TO VISUALIZE THE LONGITUDINAL OF THE BODY. NOTE THE ANTERIOR LYING STOMACH BETWEEN THE PANCREAS BODY AND LIVER. LOOK FOR THE PANCREATIC DUCT IN THE CENTER OF THE PANCREAS BODY.

● CONTINUE TO SCAN INFERIORLY THROUGH THE PANCREAS BODY UNTIL YOU ARE BEYOND IT.

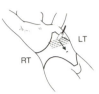

N O T E : Angling the transducer inferiorly from the midline of the body and superior to the pancreas body may aid evaluation.

● MOVE THE TRANSDUCER BACK ONTO THE PANCREAS BODY AND MOVE THE TRANSDUCER LEFT LATERAL ONTO THE PANCREAS TAIL. ROTATING THE TRANSDUCER CAN HELP VISUALIZE THE LONGITUDINAL OF THE TAIL.

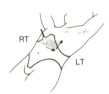

ONCE LOCATED, SCAN SUPERIORLY THROUGH THE PANCREAS TAIL UNTIL YOU ARE BEYOND IT.
● MOVE THE TRANSDUCER BACK ONTO THE TAIL AND SCAN INFERIORLY THROUGH THE PANCREAS TAIL UNTIL YOU ARE BEYOND IT.

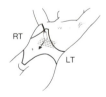

NOTE THAT THE TAIL LIES JUST POSTERIOR TO THE STOMACH AND JUST ANTERIOR TO THE LONGITUDINAL SPLENIC VEIN, WHICH IS IMMEDIATELY ANTERIOR

TO THE TRAVERSED SUPERIOR POLE OF THE LEFT KIDNEY. ALSO, IN MOST CASES THE PANCREAS TAIL IS LEFT LATERAL TO THE SUPERIOR MESENTERIC ARTERY AND AORTA. LOOK FOR THE PANCREATIC DUCT IN THE CENTER OF THE TAIL.

N O T E : Angling the transducer left lateral toward the pancreas tail from the midline of the body at the level of the pancreas body may aid evaluation. Also, using a posterior approach can aid evaluation. Look for the pancreas tail anterior to the superior pole of the left kidney.

● RETURN TO THE PANCREAS BODY AND MOVE THE TRANSDUCER RIGHT LATERAL ONTO THE PANCREAS NECK. ROTATING THE TRANSDUCER CAN HELP VISUALIZE THE LONGITUDINAL OF THE NECK. ONCE LOCATED, SCAN SUPERIORLY THROUGH THE NECK UNTIL YOU ARE BEYOND IT.

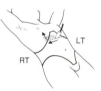

NOTE THAT THE SUPERIOR PORTION OF THE NECK LIES JUST ANTERIOR TO THE LONGITUDINAL PORTAL SPLENIC CONFLUENCE. LOOK FOR THE PANCREATIC DUCT IN THE CENTER OF THE NECK.
● MOVE BACK ONTO THE NECK AND SCAN SLIGHTLY INFERIOR THROUGH THE NECK AND ONTO THE PANCREATIC HEAD.

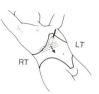

NOTE THAT THE INFERIOR PORTION OF THE NECK IS JUST ANTERIOR TO THE TRAVERSED SUPERIOR MESENTERIC VEIN THAT SEPARATES THE NECK FROM THE UNCINATE PROCESS.

NOTE: Angling the transducer right lateral toward the pancreatic neck from the midline of the body at the level of the pancreas body may aid evaluation.

● MOVE BACK ONTO THE NECK AND SCAN SLIGHTLY RIGHT LATERAL AND INFERIOR ONTO THE PANCREATIC HEAD. IF NECESSARY, ADJUST THE POSITION OF THE TRANSDUCER TO VISUALIZE BOTH SIDES OF THE HEAD, THEN CONTINUE SCANNING INFERIORLY THROUGH THE HEAD UNTIL YOU ARE BEYOND IT.

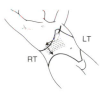

NOTE THAT THE HEAD AND UNCINATE ARE JUST ANTERIOR TO THE TRAVERSED IVC. NOTE THE TRAVERSED COMMON BILE DUCT AT THE POSTERIOR RIGHT LATERAL BORDER AND THE TRAVERSED GASTRODUODENAL ARTERY AT THE ANTERIOR RIGHT LATERAL BORDER. NOTE THE DUODENUM IMMEDIATELY RIGHT LATERAL TO THE HEAD. LOOK FOR THE PANCREATIC DUCT IN THE CENTER OF THE HEAD.

NOTE: Angling the transducer right lateral toward the pancreatic head from the midline of the body at a level inferior to the pancreatic body may aid evaluation.

TRANSVERSE SURVEY

Sagittal Plane/Anterior Approach

● BEGIN WITH THE TRANSDUCER PERPENDICULAR AND LOCATE THE DISTAL LONG AXIS PORTION OF THE IVC WHERE IT PASSES THROUGH THE LIVER. MOVE INFERIORLY ALONG THE IVC UNTIL YOU LOCATE THE HEAD OF THE PANCREAS IMMEDIATELY ANTERIOR TO IT. IN MOST CASES THIS IS AT THE LEVEL OF THE IVC WHERE THE TRAVERSED RIGHT RENAL ARTERY PASSES POSTERIOR TO IT.

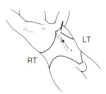

● ONCE THE PANCREAS HEAD IS LOCATED, MOVE THE TRANSDUCER RIGHT LATERAL SCANNING THROUGH THE HEAD UNTIL YOU ARE BEYOND IT. MOVE BACK ONTO THIS LATERAL PORTION OF THE HEAD AND NOTE THE TRAVERSED PORTAL VEIN AND PROPER HEPATIC ARTERY SUPERIORLY.

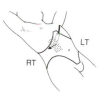

NOTE THE LONGITUDINAL COMMON BILE DUCT POSTERIORLY AND THE LONGITUDINAL GASTRODUODENAL ARTERY ANTERIORLY. NOTE THAT THE PANCREATIC HEAD LIES BETWEEN THE IVC AND THE LIVER. LOOK FOR THE PANCREATIC DUCT IN THE CENTER OF THE HEAD.

● MOVE THE TRANSDUCER SLIGHTLY TOWARD THE MIDLINE OF THE BODY AND ONTO THE UNCINATE PROCESS.

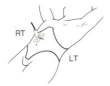

NOTE THE LONGITUDINAL SUPERIOR MESENTERIC VEIN IMMEDIATELY ANTERIOR TO THE UNCINATE SEPARATING IT FROM THE PANCREATIC NECK. IN MOST CASES THE UNCINATE LIES JUST ANTERIOR TO THE IVC, BUT IT MAY EXTEND LEFT LATERAL AND ANTERIOR TO THE AORTA.

● SCAN LEFT LATERAL THROUGH THE PANCREATIC NECK AND UNCINATE AND ONTO THE PANCREATIC BODY. IT MAY BE HELPFUL TO ROTATE THE TRANSDUCER VARYING DEGREES TO VISUALIZE THE LONG AXIS OF THE AORTA AND SUPERIOR MESENTERIC ARTERY AND LOOK FOR THE PANCREAS BODY ANTERIORLY.

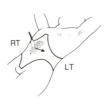

ONCE THE PANCREAS BODY IS LOCATED, NOTE THAT IT LIES IMMEDIATELY ANTERIOR TO THE TRAVERSED SPLENIC VEIN. NOTE THE TRAVERSED SPLENIC ARTERY IMMEDIATELY SUPERIOR. LOOK FOR THE PANCREATIC DUCT IN THE CENTER OF THE BODY. NOTE THE ANTERIOR AND INFERIOR LYING STOMACH BETWEEN THE PANCREAS BODY AND LIVER.

● SCAN LEFT LATERAL THROUGH AND BEYOND THE PANCREAS BODY ONTO THE PANCREAS TAIL.

NOTE THAT THE TAIL LIES JUST POSTERIOR TO THE STOMACH, JUST INFERIOR TO THE SPLENIC ARTERY, AND JUST ANTERIOR TO THE TRAVERSED SPLENIC VEIN, WHICH IS IMMEDIATELY ANTERIOR TO THE LONGITUDINAL LEFT KIDNEY. ALSO, IN MOST CASES THE TAIL LIES LEFT LATERAL TO THE AORTA. LOOK FOR THE PANCREATIC DUCT IN THE CENTER OF THE TAIL.

● CONTINUE TO SCAN LEFT LATERALLY THROUGH THE PANCREAS TAIL UNTIL YOU ARE BEYOND IT.

NOTE: Using a posterior approach can aid evaluation. Look for the pancreas tail anterior to the longitudinal left kidney.

REQUIRED PICTURES

LONGITUDINAL IMAGES

Transverse Plane/Anterior Approach

1. LONG AXIS IMAGE OF THE PANCREAS TO INCLUDE AS MUCH HEAD, UNCI-
   NATE, NECK, BODY, TAIL, AND PANCREATIC DUCT AS POSSIBLE.

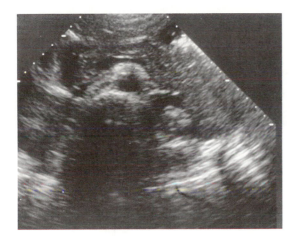 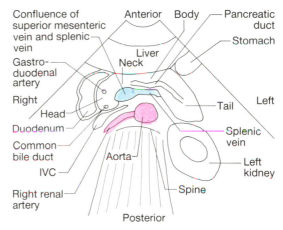

LABELED: PANCREAS TRV LONG AXIS

2. LONGITUDINAL IMAGE OF THE PANCREAS BODY AND NECK TO INCLUDE THE SPLENIC VEIN.

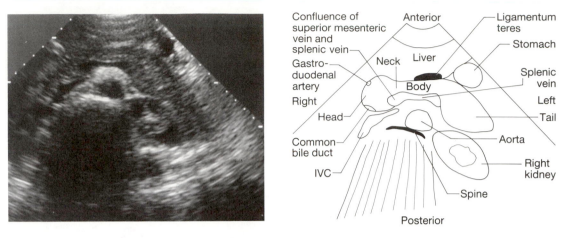

LABELED: PANCREAS TRV BODY/NECK

3. LONGITUDINAL IMAGE OF THE PANCREAS TAIL.

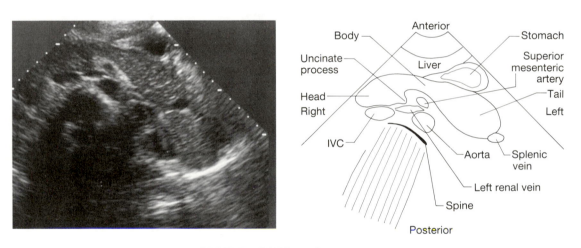

LABELED: PANCREAS TRV TAIL

4. LONGITUDINAL IMAGE OF THE PANCREAS HEAD TO INCLUDE THE UNCI-
    NATE PROCESS AND COMMON BILE DUCT (IF BILE-FILLED).

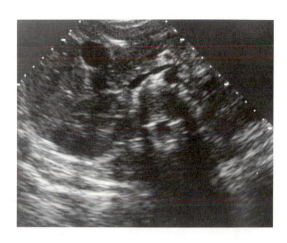 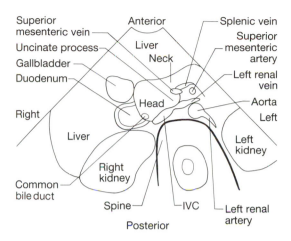

LABELED: PANCREAS TRV HEAD

TRANSVERSE IMAGES

Sagittal Plane/Anterior Approach

5. TRANSVERSE IMAGE OF THE PANCREAS HEAD TO INCLUDE THE COMMON
    BILE DUCT (IF BILE-FILLED).

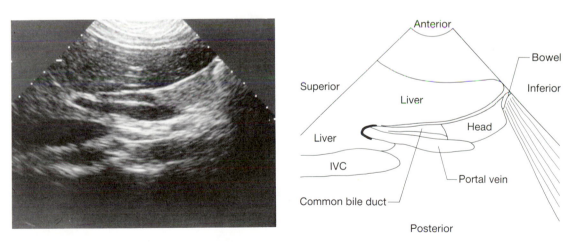

LABELED: PANCREAS SAG HEAD

6. TRANSVERSE IMAGE OF THE PANCREAS NECK AND UNCINATE PROCESS TO INCLUDE THE SUPERIOR MESENTERIC VEIN.

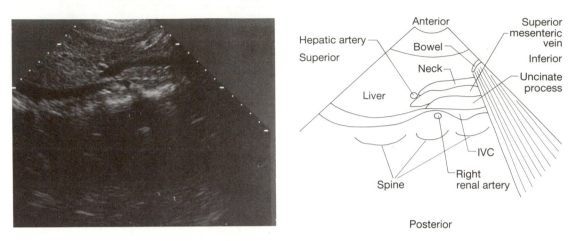

LABELED: PANCREAS SAG NECK/UNCINATE

7. TRANSVERSE IMAGE OF THE PANCREAS BODY TO INCLUDE THE SPLENIC VEIN.

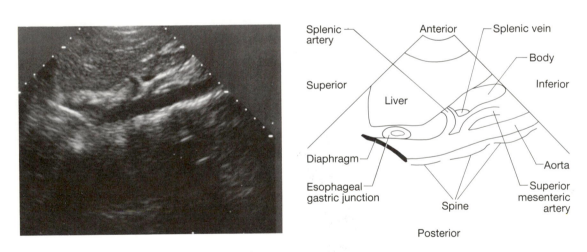

LABELED: PANCREAS SAG BODY

8. TRANSVERSE IMAGE OF THE PANCREAS TAIL.

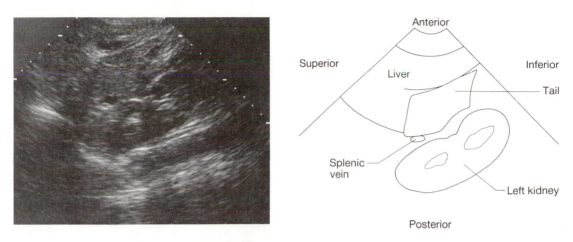

LABELED: PANCREAS SAG TAIL

NOTE: Measurements of the normal pancreas are not required.

NOTE: If the pancreas cannot be seen because of overlying bowel gas, and the patient cannot be given fluids and every effort has been made to image the pancreas, take the above images in the designated area and add "area" to the labeling.

REQUIRED PICTURES WHEN THE PANCREAS IS NOT THE PRIMARY AREA OF INTEREST

LONGITUDINAL IMAGES

Transverse Plane/Anterior Approach

1. LONG AXIS IMAGE OF THE PANCREAS TO INCLUDE AS MUCH HEAD, UNCI-NATE, NECK, BODY, TAIL, AND PANCREATIC DUCT AS POSSIBLE.

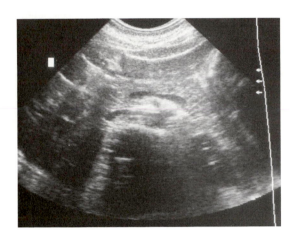 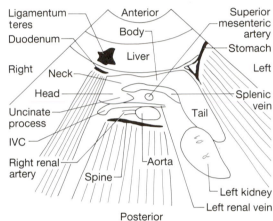

LABELED: PANCREAS TRV LONG AXIS

2. LONGITUDINAL IMAGE OF THE PANCREAS HEAD TO INCLUDE THE UNCINATE PROCESS AND COMMON BILE DUCT (IF BILE-FILLED).

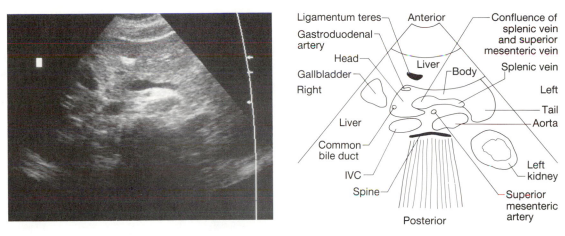

LABELED: PANCREAS TRV HEAD

TRANSVERSE IMAGE

Sagittal Plane/Anterior Approach

3. TRANSVERSE IMAGE OF THE PANCREAS HEAD TO INCLUDE THE COMMON BILE DUCT (IF BILE-FILLED).

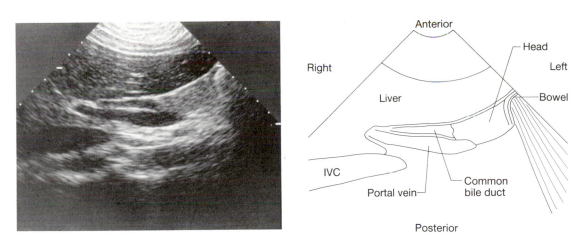

LABELED: PANCREAS SAG HEAD

NOTE: If the pancreas cannot be seen because of overlying bowel gas and the patient cannot be given fluids and every effort has been made to image the pancreas, take the above images in the designated areas and add "area" to the labeling.

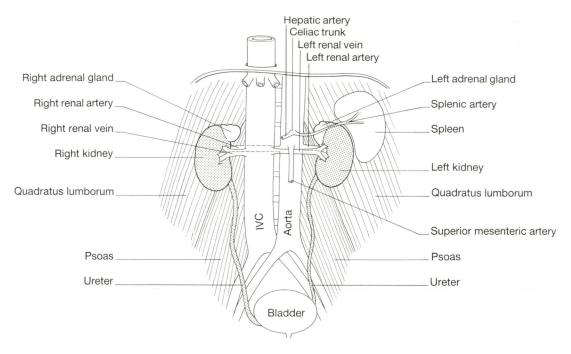

Hepatic artery
Celiac trunk
Left renal vein
Left renal artery

Right adrenal gland

Right renal artery

Right renal vein

Right kidney

Quadratus lumborum

IVC

Aorta

Psoas

Ureter

Bladder

Left adrenal gland

Splenic artery

Spleen

Left kidney

Quadratus lumborum

Superior mesenteric artery

Psoas

Ureter

Location of the urinary system

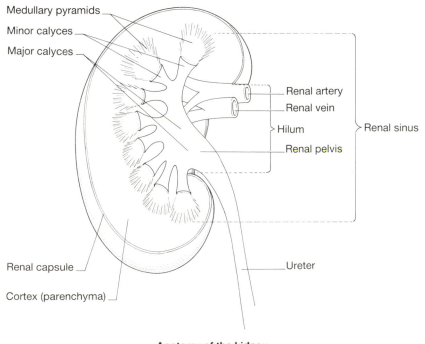

Medullary pyramids

Minor calyces

Major calyces

Renal artery

Renal vein

Hilum

Renal pelvis

Renal sinus

Renal capsule

Cortex (parenchyma)

Ureter

Anatomy of the kidney

CHAPTER TEN
RENAL SCANNING PROTOCOL

LOCATION

- The kidneys lie on each side of the spine in the area between the 12th thoracic and 4th lumbar vertebrae.

- Retroperitoneal.

- The right kidney is lower than the left kidney.

- The right kidney is posteroinferior to the liver and gallbladder.

- The left kidney is inferior and medial to the spleen.

- The kidneys lie immediately anterior to the psoas and quadratus lumborum muscles.

- Located superior, anterior, and medial to each kidney is the adrenal gland.

ANATOMY

- The kidneys are covered by a fibrous "renal or true capsule."

- Fat surrounds the encapsulated kidneys in the perinephric space.

- Gerota's fascia is a fibrous sheath that encloses each kidney, perinephric fat, and adrenal gland.

- Normal adult kidneys are 9 to 12 cm long, 2.5 to 3.5 cm thick, and 4 to 5 cm wide.

- The kidneys are composed of two distinct areas:

  - Sinus:
    The entrance to the sinus is referred to as the hilum. Through it passes the renal arteries, veins, nerves, lymphatic vessels, and ureter.
    The sinus contains fat and the renal pelvis, which is formed by the expanded superior end of the ureter. The renal pelvis is a urine reservoir or collecting system that divides into the infundibula: two or three major calyces that in turn divide into 8 or 18 minor calyces. Each minor calyx is indented by the top or apex of a medullary pyramid, which it receives urine from.

Parenchyma:

Surrounds the sinus.

Outer cortex:

Contains millions of nephrons, the microscopic functional units of the kidney. Site of urine formation. The cortex lies between the renal capsule and the medulla.

Inner medulla:

Consists of 8 to 18 renal pyramids that pass urine to the minor calyces. The bases of the pyramids form a margin with the cortex. The apices of the pyramids project into the bottom or side of the renal sinus and into the minor calyces. The pyramids are separated from each other by bands of cortical tissue referred to as the columns of Bertin, which extend inward to the renal sinus.

PHYSIOLOGY

- As part of the excretory system, kidneys function to get rid of metabolic wastes.

- Kidneys purify the blood by excreting urine (excess water, salt, toxins).

SONOGRAPHIC APPEARANCE

- Because of the fat, the renal sinus is echogenic with variable contour. Parenchyma surrounds the sinus.

- The infundibula and renal pelvis are not seen if collapsed, otherwise they appear anechoic.

- The cortex is midgray or medium- to low-level echoes with even texture that is less echogenic than the normal liver or spleen. The contour of the normal cortex should appear smooth. The cortex is surrounded by the echogenic renal capsule.

- The medullary pyramids appear as triangular, round, or blunted hypoechoic areas to the more urine-filled anechoic areas.

- Arcuate vessels can be seen at the corticomedullary junction as echogenic dots.

- The ureters are not normally seen.

NORMAL VARIANTS

- Dromedary humps:

  - Cortical bulge(s) on the lateral border of the kidney.

  - Sonographic appearance is the same as normal renal cortex.

- Hypertrophied column of Bertin:

  - At varying degrees of size, cortical tissue indents the renal sinus.

  - Sonographic appearance is the same as normal renal cortex.

- Double collecting system:

  - The renal sinus is divided by a hypertrophied column of Bertin.

  - Sonographic appearance is the same as normal renal cortex and normal renal sinus.

- Horseshoe kidney:

  - The kidneys are connected, usually at the lower poles.

  - Sonographic appearance is the same as normal renal cortex.

- Renal ectopia:
  - One or both kidneys may be found outside the normal renal fossa.
  - Other locations include lower abdominal to pelvic and rarely intrathoracic.

PATIENT PREP

- None.

PATIENT POSITION

RIGHT KIDNEY

- **Supine.**
- Left posterior oblique, left lateral decubitus, and prone as needed.

LEFT KIDNEY

- **Right lateral decubitus.**
- Prone as needed.

NOTE: Different patient positions should be used whenever the suggested position does not give the desired results.

TRANSDUCER

- **3.0 MHz** or **3.5 MHz.**
- 5.0 MHz for very thin patient.

BREATHING TECHNIQUE

- **Deep, held inspiration.**

RENAL SURVEY

NOTE: While surveying the kidneys, evaluate the perirenal regions for possible abnormalities.

RIGHT KIDNEY SURVEY

Longitudinal Survey

Sagittal Plane/Anterior Approach

● BEGIN WITH THE TRANSDUCER PER-PENDICULAR, JUST INFERIOR TO THE MOST LATERAL EDGE OF THE RIGHT COSTAL MARGIN.

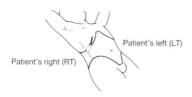

Patient's left (LT)

Patient's right (RT)

● IF THE KIDNEY IS NOT SEEN HERE, MOVE THE TRANSDUCER IN MEDIAL AND INFERIOR SECTIONS UNTIL THE KIDNEY IS LOCATED.

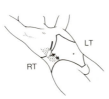

● ONCE THE KIDNEY IS LOCATED, RO-TATE THE TRANSDUCER AT VARYING DE-GREES (TO OBLIQUE THE SCANNING PLANE ACCORDING TO THE LIE OF THE RIGHT KIDNEY) TO VISUALIZE THE LONG AXIS OF THE KIDNEY.

● ONCE THE LONG AXIS IS LOCATED, SLIGHTLY ROCK THE TRANSDUCER RIGHT TO LEFT AND SLIDE THE TRANS-DUCER MEDIALLY SCANNING THROUGH THE KIDNEY UNTIL YOU ARE BEYOND IT.

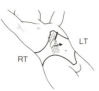

● MOVE BACK ONTO THE MEDIAL POR-TION OF THE KIDNEY. ROCKING AND SLID-ING, SCAN THROUGH THE LATERAL POR-TION OF THE KIDNEY UNTIL YOU ARE BEYOND IT.

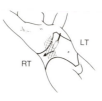

NOTE: Longitudinal survey of the right kidney can be performed from a coronal plane, right lateral approach. Begin with the transducer perpendicular, midcoronal plane, just superior to the iliac crest. Move or angle the transducer superior to inferior or scan intercostal if necessary to locate the kidney.

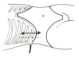

Follow the above scanning methods. Note that this approach is generally easier when the patient is in the left lateral decubitus position.

Transverse Survey

Transverse Plane/Anterior Approach

● STILL IN THE SAGITTAL SCANNING PLANE, LOCATE THE LONG AXIS OF THE RIGHT KIDNEY. ROTATE THE TRANSDUCER 90 DEGREES INTO THE TRANSVERSE SCANNING PLANE AND TRAVERSE THE KIDNEY.

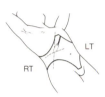

NOTE: Alternatively, begin the transverse survey in the transverse plane with the transducer perpendicular, just inferior to the costal margin of the medial angle of the ribs. Move the transducer in right lateral and inferior sections until the kidney is located.

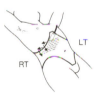

● ONCE THE KIDNEY IS LOCATED, MOVE THE TRANSDUCER SLIGHTLY SUPERIOR AND MEDIAL TO INFERIOR AND LATERAL TO FIND THE MIDPORTION AND HILUM OF THE KIDNEY. SLIGHT AND VARYING DEGREES OF TRANSDUCER OBLIQUES MAY BE NECESSARY TO RESOLVE THE HILUM. NOTE THE RENAL ARTERY AND VEIN.

- FROM THE HILUM, SLIGHTLY ROCK THE TRANSDUCER SUPERIOR TO INFERIOR AND AT THE SAME TIME SLIDE THE TRANSDUCER SUPERIOR AND MEDIAL THROUGH AND BEYOND THE SUPERIOR POLE OF THE KIDNEY.

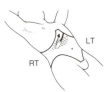

- CONTINUE ROCKING, AND MOVE THE TRANSDUCER BACK ONTO THE SUPERIOR POLE. SLIDE THE TRANSDUCER INFERIOR AND LATERAL THROUGH MIDKIDNEY AND THE INFERIOR POLE. SCAN THROUGH AND BEYOND THE INFERIOR POLE.

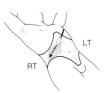

NOTE: Transverse survey of the right kidney can be performed from a right lateral approach. Use the same scanning approach mentioned for the coronal longitudinal survey and follow the above scanning methods.

LEFT KIDNEY SURVEY

Longitudinal Survey

Coronal Plane/Left Lateral Approach

NOTE: Although this approach can be performed with the patient supine, it is generally easier with the patient in the right lateral decubitus position. Imaging quality might be improved by placing a sponge or rolled towel under the patient's right side. This opens up the rib spaces.

- BEGIN WITH THE TRANSDUCER PERPENDICULAR, MIDCORONAL PLANE, JUST SUPERIOR TO THE ILIAC CREST.

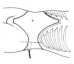

NOTE: If the kidney is not seen in the midcoronal plane, try approaches just to the right and left of the midline.

● MOVE OR ANGLE THE TRANSDUCER SUPERIOR TO INFERIOR TO LOCATE THE KIDNEY. ONCE LOCATED, ROTATE THE TRANSDUCER AT VARYING DEGREES (TO OBLIQUE THE SCANNING PLANE ACCORDING TO THE LIE OF THE LEFT KIDNEY) TO VISUALIZE THE LONG AXIS OF THE KIDNEY.

● ONCE THE LONG AXIS IS LOCATED, SLIGHTLY ROCK THE TRANSDUCER SIDE TO SIDE AND AT THE SAME TIME SLIDE THE TRANSDUCER TOWARD THE PATIENT'S FRONT, SCANNING THROUGH THE ANTERIOR PORTION OF THE KIDNEY UNTIL YOU ARE BEYOND IT.

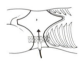

● MOVE BACK ONTO THE ANTERIOR PORTION OF THE KIDNEY. ROCKING AND SLIDING, MOVE TOWARD THE PATIENT'S BACK, SCANNING THROUGH THE POSTERIOR PORTION OF THE KIDNEY UNTIL YOU ARE BEYOND IT.

NOTE: Longitudinal survey of the left kidney may have to be performed intercostally, depending on body habitus and the position of the kidney. Begin with the transducer perpendicular, midcoronal plane, in the first inferior intercostal space. Move to the adjacent intercostal spaces to evaluate the entire kidney. Varying respiration and angling the transducer within the intercostal spaces can aid evaluation. In some cases, only the superior pole will have to be evaluated intercostally.

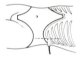

Transverse Survey

Transverse Plane/Left Lateral Approach

• STILL IN THE CORONAL SCANNING PLANE, LOCATE THE LONG AXIS OF THE LEFT KIDNEY. ROTATE THE TRANSDUCER 90 DEGREES INTO THE TRANSVERSE SCANNING PLANE AND TRAVERSE THE KIDNEY.

NOTE: Alternatively, begin the transverse survey in the transverse plane with the transducer perpendicular, just superior to the iliac crest. Move or angle the transducer superior to inferior to locate the kidney.

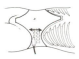

• ONCE THE KIDNEY IS LOCATED, MOVE THE TRANSDUCER SUPERIOR TO INFERIOR TO FIND THE MIDPORTION AND HILUM OF THE KIDNEY. SLIGHT AND VARYING DEGREES OF TRANSDUCER OBLIQUES MAY BE NECESSARY TO RESOLVE THE HILUM.

NOTE THE RENAL ARTERY AND VEIN.
• FROM THE HILUM, SLIGHTLY ROCK THE TRANSDUCER SUPERIOR TO INFERIOR AND AT THE SAME TIME SLIDE THE TRANSDUCER SUPERIOR THROUGH AND BEYOND THE SUPERIOR POLE OF THE KIDNEY.

• CONTINUE ROCKING AND MOVE THE TRANSDUCER BACK ONTO THE SUPERIOR POLE. SLIDE THE TRANSDUCER INFERIOR THROUGH THE MIDKIDNEY AND THE INFERIOR POLE. SCAN THROUGH AND BEYOND THE INFERIOR POLE.

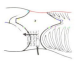

NOTE: Transverse survey of the left kidney may have to be performed intercostally. Use the same approach mentioned for the intercostal coronal longitudinal survey and follow the above scanning methods.

REQUIRED PICTURES

RIGHT KIDNEY

Longitudinal Images

Sagittal Plane/Anterior Approach

1. LONG AXIS IMAGE OF THE RIGHT KIDNEY WITH *SUPERIOR TO INFERIOR MEASUREMENT*.

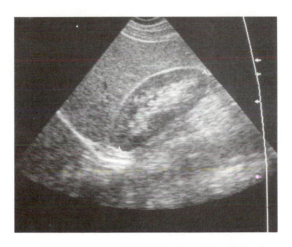

LABELED: RT KIDNEY SAG LONG AXIS

2. SAME IMAGE AS NUMBER 1 WITHOUT CALIPERS.

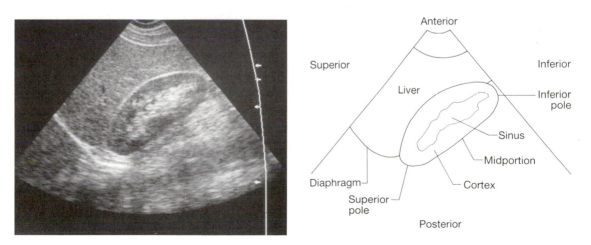

LABELED: RT KIDNEY SAG LONG AXIS

3. LONG AXIS IMAGE OF THE RIGHT KIDNEY WITH *SUPERIOR TO INFERIOR MEASUREMENT*.

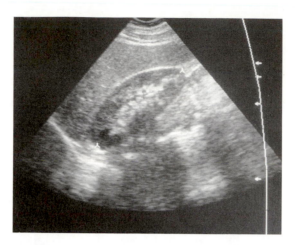

LABELED: RT KIDNEY SAG LONG AXIS

4. SAME IMAGE AS NUMBER 3 WITHOUT CALIPERS.

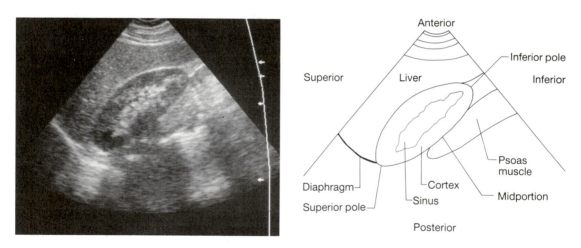

LABELED: RT KIDNEY SAG LONG AXIS

NOTE: In many cases superior and/or inferior pole definition is sacrificed to achieve the long axis. If so, take those images here and label accordingly.

5. LONGITUDINAL IMAGE OF THE RIGHT KIDNEY SUPERIOR POLE.

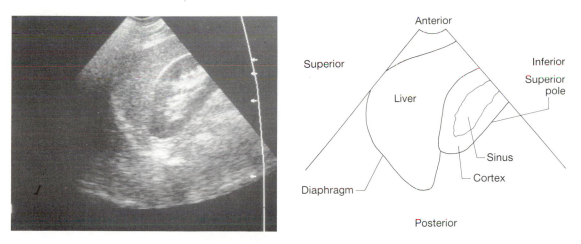

LABELED: RT KIDNEY SAG SUP POLE

6. LONGITUDINAL IMAGE OF THE RIGHT KIDNEY INFERIOR POLE.

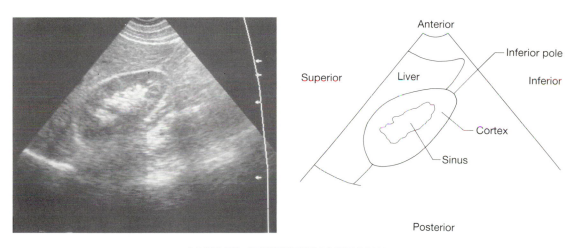

LABELED: RT KIDNEY SAG INF POLE

7. LONGITUDINAL IMAGE OF THE RIGHT KIDNEY JUST MEDIAL TO THE LONG AXIS.

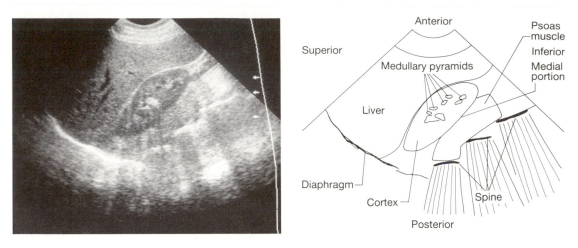

LABELED: RT KIDNEY SAG MED

8. LONGITUDINAL IMAGE OF THE RIGHT KIDNEY JUST LATERAL TO THE LONG AXIS TO INCLUDE PART OF THE LIVER FOR PARENCHYMA COMPARISON.

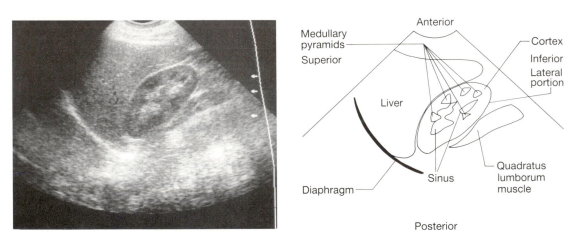

LABELED: RT KIDNEY SAG LAT

Transverse Images

Transverse Plane/Anterior Approach

9. TRANSVERSE IMAGE OF THE RIGHT KIDNEY SUPERIOR POLE.

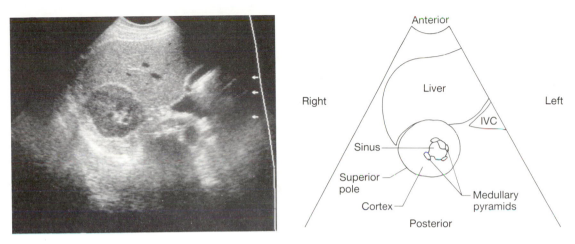

LABELED: RT KIDNEY TRV SUP POLE

10. TRANSVERSE IMAGE OF THE RIGHT KIDNEY MIDPORTION TO INCLUDE THE HILUM WITH *ANTERIOR TO POSTERIOR MEASUREMENT*.

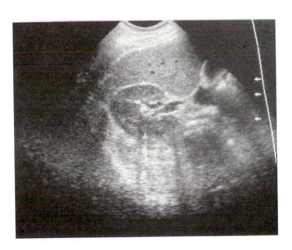

LABELED: RT KIDNEY TRV MID

11. SAME IMAGE AS NUMBER 10 WITHOUT CALIPERS.

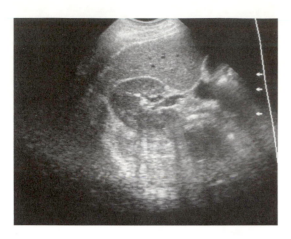
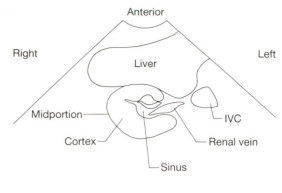

LABELED: RT KIDNEY TRV MID

If see liver it's upper pole
no liver lower pole

12. TRANSVERSE IMAGE OF THE RIGHT KIDNEY INFERIOR POLE.

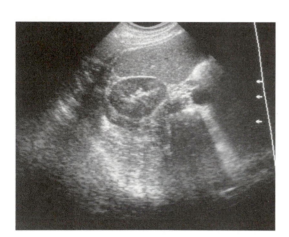
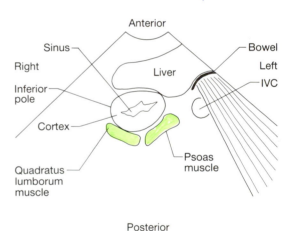

LABELED: RT KIDNEY TRV INF POLE

LEFT KIDNEY

Longitudinal Images

Coronal Plane/Left Lateral Approach

1. LONG AXIS IMAGE OF THE LEFT KIDNEY WITH *SUPERIOR TO INFERIOR MEASUREMENT*.

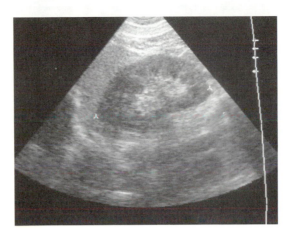

LABELED: LT KIDNEY COR LONG AXIS

2. SAME IMAGE AS NUMBER 1 WITHOUT CALIPERS.

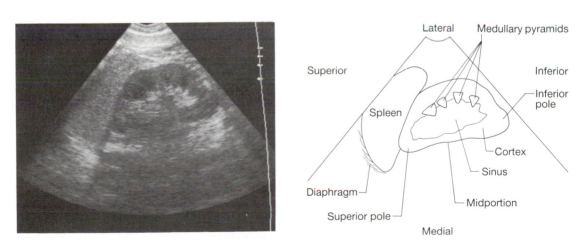

LABELED: LT KIDNEY COR LONG AXIS

Coronal view

3. LONG AXIS IMAGE OF THE LEFT KIDNEY WITH *SUPERIOR TO INFERIOR MEASUREMENT*.

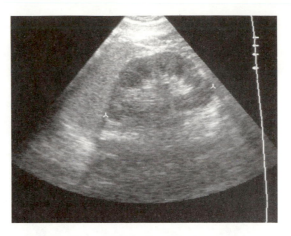

LABELED: LT KIDNEY COR LONG AXIS

4. SAME IMAGE AS NUMBER 3 WITHOUT CALIPERS.

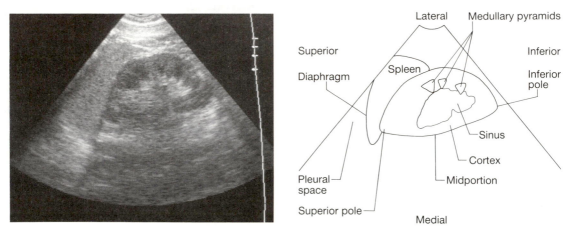

LABELED: LT KIDNEY COR LONG AXIS

NOTE: In many cases, superior and/or inferior pole definition is sacrificed to achieve the long axis. If so, take those images here and label accordingly.

NOTE: One of the long axis images or, if applicable, the superior pole image must include part of the spleen for parenchyma comparison.

5. LONGITUDINAL IMAGE OF THE LEFT KIDNEY SUPERIOR POLE.

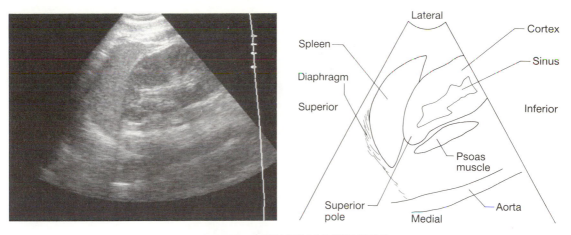

LABELED: LT KIDNEY COR SUP POLE

6. LONGITUDINAL IMAGE OF THE LEFT KIDNEY INFERIOR POLE.

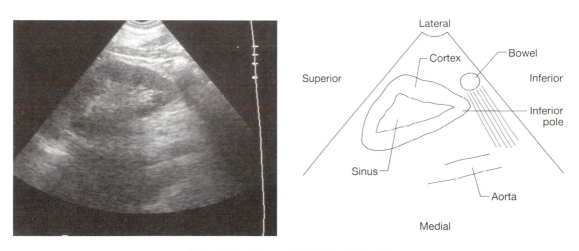

LABELED: LT KIDNEY COR INF POLE

7. LONGITUDINAL IMAGE OF THE LEFT KIDNEY JUST ANTERIOR TO THE LONG AXIS.

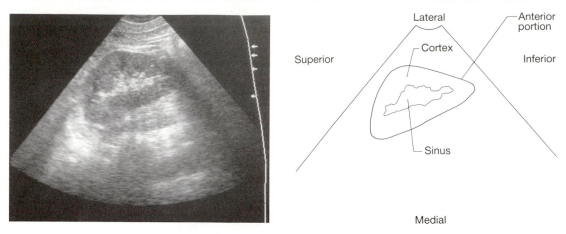

LABELED: LT KIDNEY COR ANT

Dromedary hump = normal varient of left kidney

8. LONGITUDINAL IMAGE OF THE LEFT KIDNEY JUST POSTERIOR TO THE LONG AXIS.

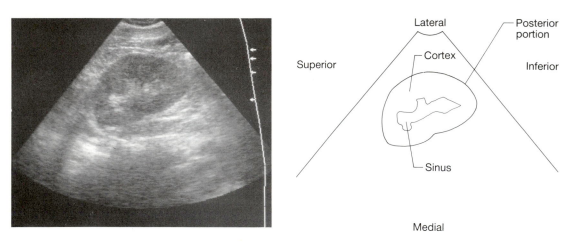

LABELED: LT KIDNEY COR POST

Transverse Images

Transverse Plane/Left Lateral Approach

9. TRANSVERSE IMAGE OF THE LEFT KIDNEY SUPERIOR POLE.

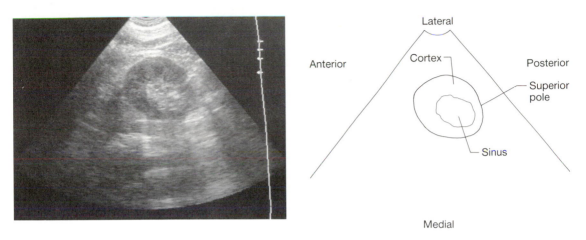

LABELED: LT KIDNEY LT TRV SUP POLE

10. TRANSVERSE IMAGE OF THE LEFT KIDNEY MIDPORTION TO INCLUDE THE HILUM WITH *ANTERIOR TO POSTERIOR MEASUREMENT*.

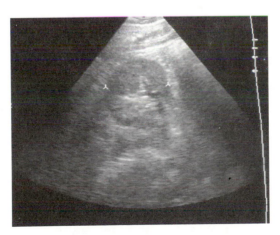

LABELED: LT KIDNEY LT TRV MID

11. SAME IMAGE AS NUMBER 10 WITHOUT CALIPERS.

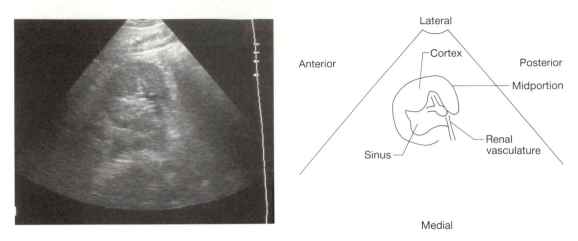

LABELED: LT KIDNEY LT TRV MID

12. TRANSVERSE IMAGE OF THE LEFT KIDNEY INFERIOR POLE.

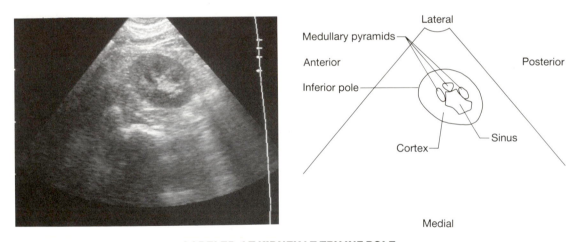

LABELED: LT KIDNEY LT TRV INF POLE

REQUIRED PICTURES WHEN THE KIDNEYS ARE NOT THE PRIMARY AREA OF INTEREST

RIGHT KIDNEY

Longitudinal Image(s)

Sagittal Plane/Anterior Approach

1. LONG AXIS IMAGE OF THE RIGHT KIDNEY.

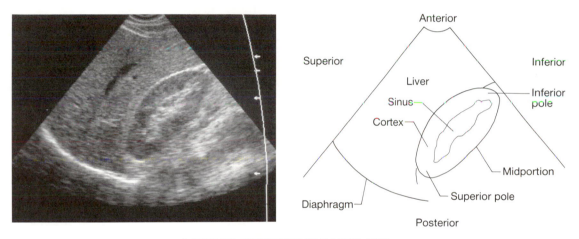

LABELED: RT KIDNEY SAG LONG AXIS

NOTE: Take additional images of the superior and/or inferior poles if they are not clearly defined and label accordingly.

Transverse Image

Transverse Plane/Anterior Approach

2. TRANSVERSE IMAGE OF THE RIGHT KIDNEY MIDPORTION TO INCLUDE THE HILUM.

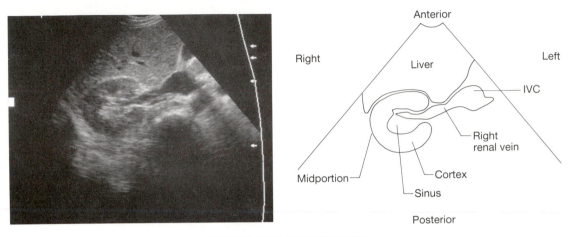

LABELED: RT KIDNEY TRV MID

LEFT KIDNEY

Longitudinal Image(s)

Coronal Plane/Left Lateral Approach

3. LONG AXIS IMAGE OF THE LEFT KIDNEY.

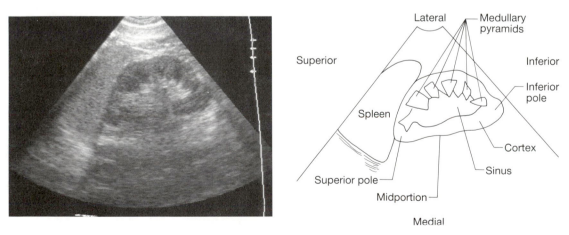

LABELED: LT KIDNEY COR LONG AXIS

NOTE: Take additional images of the superior and/or inferior poles if they are not clearly defined and label accordingly.

Transverse Image

Transverse Plane/Left Lateral Approach

4. TRANSVERSE IMAGE OF THE LEFT KIDNEY MIDPORTION TO INCLUDE THE HILUM.

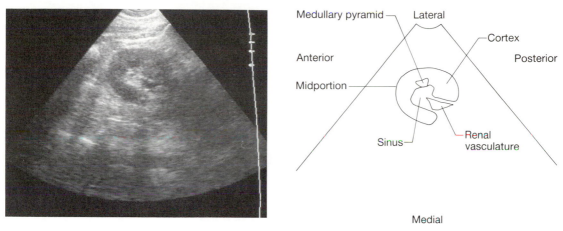

LABELED: LT KIDNEY LT TRV MID

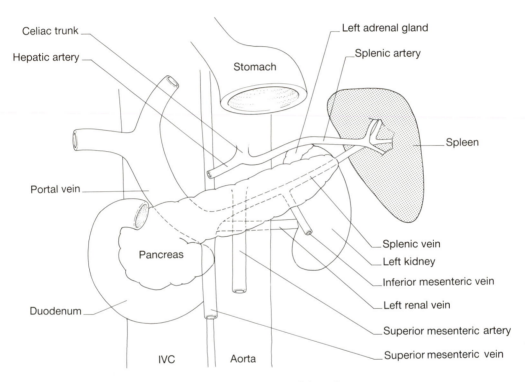

Location and anatomy of the spleen

Celiac trunk

Hepatic artery

Stomach

Left adrenal gland

Splenic artery

Spleen

Portal vein

Pancreas

Splenic vein

Left kidney

Inferior mesenteric vein

Left renal vein

Superior mesenteric artery

Duodenum

Superior mesenteric vein

IVC

Aorta

118

CHAPTER ELEVEN
SPLEEN SCANNING PROTOCOL

LOCATION

- Occupies the posterolateral section of the left upper quadrant.

- Intraperitoneal (except for its hilum).

- Immediately inferior and anterior to the diaphragm.

- Lateral to the stomach and, depending on its size, sometimes posterior to it.

- Lateral to the tail of the pancreas, left kidney, adrenal gland, and the splenic flexure of the colon.

ANATOMY

- Size is variable but is considered normal when it appears about the same size as the adjacent left kidney.

- Shape is variable but may resemble a half moon.

- The splenic vein and artery, lymphatic vessels, and nerves pass through the splenic hilum.

- The splenic vein passes through the splenic hilum and courses immediately posterior to the tail and body of the pancreas to join the superior mesenteric vein posterior to the pancreas neck to form the portal vein.

- The splenic artery courses from the celiac trunk of the aorta immediately superior to the body and tail of the pancreas to enter the splenic hilum.

PHYSIOLOGY

- The spleen is a large mass of lymphatic tissue that is part of the reticuloendothelial system.

- Although not essential to life, the spleen filters foreign material from the blood, and forms antibodies. It also breaks down hemoglobin, is a blood reservoir, and is important for blood formation in the fetus or when there is severe anemia.

SONOGRAPHIC APPEARANCE

- The parenchyma of the spleen is mid-gray or medium-level echoes with even texture that is usually the same as the normal liver but may appear slightly less echogenic.

- Interspersed within the spleen are small vascular structures that are seen as branching, anechoic, and round or tubular. Closer to the hilum the larger venous structures can be distinguished from the smaller arterial branches.

- The outer contour of the normal spleen should appear smooth.

NORMAL VARIANTS

- Accessory spleen:
  - Splenic tissue found separate from the organ.
  - Found most often at the splenic hilum.
  - Sonographic appearance is the same as normal splenic tissue.
- Asplenia:
  - Rare absence of the spleen.
  - Often associated with congestive heart disease.

PATIENT PREP

- None.

PATIENT POSITION

- **Right lateral decubitus.**
- Supine, sitting semierect to erect and prone as needed.

NOTE: Different patient positions should be used whenever the suggested position does not give the desired results.

TRANSDUCER

- **5.0 MHz** for intercostal or lateral subcostal scanning approaches.
- 3.0 or 3.5 MHz for anterior or posterior scanning approaches.

BREATHING TECHNIQUE

- **Deep, held inspiration.**

NOTE: Different breathing techniques should be used whenever the suggested breathing technique does not give the desired results.

SPLEEN SURVEY

LONGITUDINAL SURVEY

Coronal Plane/Left Lateral Approach

NOTE: Although this approach can be performed with the patient supine, it is generally easier with the patient in the right lateral decubitus position. Imaging quality might be improved by placing a sponge or rolled towel under the patient's right side. This opens up the rib spaces.

- BEGIN WITH THE TRANSDUCER PERPENDICULAR, MIDCORONAL PLANE, IN THE MOST INFERIOR INTERCOSTAL SPACE. IN MOST CASES THE SUPERIOR AND INFERIOR MARGINS OF THE SPLEEN CAN BE VISUALIZED FROM THIS SPACE. HOW MUCH OF THE NORMAL SPLEEN YOU SEE, HOWEVER, WILL DEPEND ON ITS SHAPE AND BODY HABITUS. IF THE SPLEEN IS NOT SEEN IN THE INFERIOR INTERCOSTAL SPACE, MOVE TO ADJACENT SUPERIOR INTERCOSTAL SPACES.

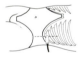

- ONCE THE SPLEEN IS LOCATED, ROTATE THE TRANSDUCER AT VARYING DEGREES (TO OBLIQUE THE SCANNING PLANE ACCORDING TO THE LIE OF THE SPLEEN) TO VISUALIZE THE LONG AXIS OF THE SPLEEN.

  NOTE THE ADJACENT PLEURAL SPACE SUPERIORLY AND THE LEFT KIDNEY AND PERINEPHRIC SPACE INFERIORLY. THE SPLENIC HILUM MAY ALSO BE SEEN MEDIALLY. SLIGHTLY ROTATING THE TRANSDUCER CAN AID EVALUATION OF THE HILUM.

• WHILE VISUALIZING THE LONG AXIS OF THE SPLEEN, MOVE OR ANGLE THE TRANSDUCER WITHIN THE INTERCOSTAL SPACE TOWARD THE PATIENT'S FRONT, SCANNING THROUGH THE ANTERIOR PORTION OF THE SPLEEN UNTIL YOU ARE BEYOND IT.

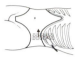

• MOVE BACK ONTO THE SPLEEN AND MOVE OR ANGLE THE TRANSDUCER TOWARD THE PATIENT'S BACK, SCANNING THROUGH THE POSTERIOR PORTION OF THE SPLEEN UNTIL YOU ARE BEYOND IT.

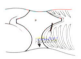

NOTE: Rib shadows are a consequence of intercostal scanning and may obscure part of the spleen. In most cases, angling the transducer within the intercostal space toward the unseen area or moving to an adjacent rib space will aid visualization.

TRANSVERSE SURVEY

Transverse Plane/Left Lateral Approach

• STILL IN THE CORONAL SCANNING PLANE, LOCATE THE LONG AXIS OF THE SPLEEN, THEN ROTATE THE TRANSDUCER 90 DEGREES INTO THE TRANSVERSE SCANNING PLANE AND TRAVERSE THE SPLEEN. NOTE THE ANTERIOR AND POSTERIOR MARGINS OF THE SPLEEN AND THE SPLENIC HILUM MEDIALLY.

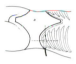

• MOVE OR ANGLE THE TRANSDUCER SUPERIORLY, SCANNING THROUGH THE SUPERIOR PORTION OF THE SPLEEN UNTIL YOU ARE BEYOND IT. NOTE THE ADJACENT PLEURAL SPACE.

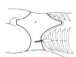

• MOVE BACK ONTO THE SPLEEN AND MOVE OR ANGLE THE TRANSDUCER INFERIORLY, SCANNING THROUGH THE INFERIOR PORTION OF THE SPLEEN UNTIL YOU ARE BEYOND IT.

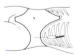

REQUIRED PICTURES

LONGITUDINAL IMAGES

Coronal Plane/Left Lateral Approach

1. LONG AXIS IMAGE OF THE SPLEEN.

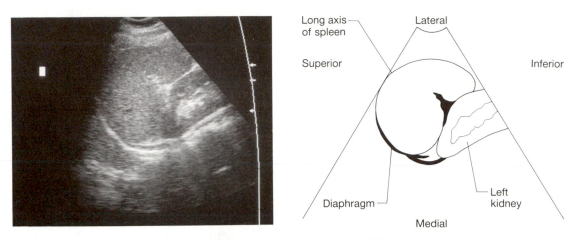

LABELED: SPLEEN COR LONG AXIS

2. SUPERIOR LONGITUDINAL IMAGE OF THE SPLEEN TO INCLUDE THE ADJACENT PLEURAL SPACE.

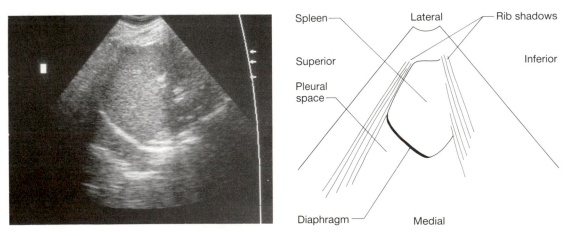

LABELED: SPLEEN COR SUP

3. INFERIOR LONGITUDINAL IMAGE OF THE SPLEEN TO INCLUDE PART OF THE LEFT KIDNEY FOR PARENCHYMA COMPARISON.

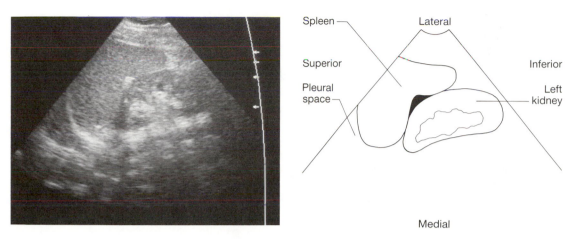

LABELED: SPLEEN COR INF

TRANSVERSE IMAGES

Transverse Plane/Left Lateral Approach

4. TRANSVERSE IMAGE OF THE SPLEEN TO INCLUDE BOTH ANTERIOR AND POSTERIOR MARGINS.

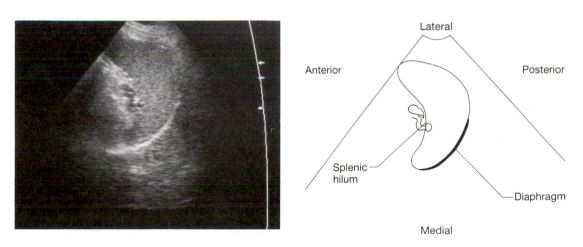

LABELED: SPLEEN LT TRV

5. TRANSVERSE IMAGE OF THE SPLEEN TO INCLUDE THE ANTERIOR MARGIN AND SPLENIC HILUM.

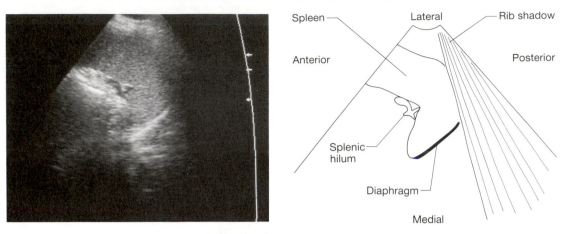

LABELED: SPLEEN LT TRV ANT

6. TRANSVERSE IMAGE OF THE SPLEEN TO INCLUDE THE POSTERIOR MARGIN.

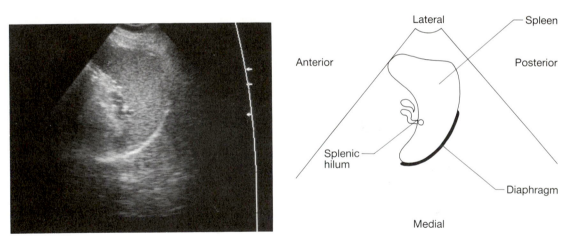

LABELED: SPLEEN LT TRV POST

REQUIRED PICTURES WHEN THE SPLEEN IS NOT THE PRIMARY AREA OF INTEREST

REQUIRED PICTURES ARE THE SAME AS THE ABOVE EXCEPT THAT:

1. THE LONGITUDINAL IMAGES OF THE SPLEEN THAT INCLUDE THE ADJACENT PLEURAL SPACE AND PART OF THE LEFT KIDNEY MAY BE COMBINED INTO ONE IMAGE IF ALL OF THE STRUCTURES ARE CLEARLY SEEN. LABEL THE IMAGE: **SPLEEN COR.** IN SOME CASES THESE STRUCTURES MAY ALSO BE SEEN ON THE LONG AXIS IMAGE. IF SO, LABEL THE IMAGE: **SPLEEN LONG AXIS.**

2. ONLY ONE TRANSVERSE IMAGE OF THE SPLEEN IS NECESSARY AS LONG AS THE ANTERIOR AND POSTERIOR MARGINS OF THE SPLEEN ARE WELL VISUALIZED.

LABEL THE IMAGE: SPLEEN LT. TRV.

PART III

PELVIC SCANNING PROTOCOLS

CHAPTER TWELVE
PELVIC SCANNING PROTOCOLS OVERVIEW

STANDARD

- No single-organ examinations. The total pelvic cavity is evaluated.
- Protocols give image specifics.
- Use real-time transabdominal or endocavital scanners with sector or curved linear transducers.

SURVEY

- Exams begin with a survey of the pelvic cavity and organs in two scanning planes.
- The transverse survey extends from the symphysis pubis to the umbilicus.
- The longitudinal survey extends from one side of the pelvic cavity to the other side.
- Protocols give survey specifications.
- Do not take any images during the survey. The survey is used to determine the correct technique, presence or lack of pathology, and the recognition of any normal variants.
- If pathology is seen, it is surveyed after the pelvic cavity and organs in two scanning planes.

CONSIDERATIONS

- Sonographic patterns in the pelvic cavity:
  - Organs, muscles, and tissues: echo texture.

  - Blood vessels, fluid-filled urinary bladder, and ovarian follicles: anechoic with echogenic walls.
  - GI tract: hypoechoic walls, varying degrees of echogenic (gas) to hypoechoic (fluid) centers.
  - Endometrial cavity and vaginal canal: echogenic to hypoechoic.
  - Bone: echogenic.
- Verbal or written consent from the patient is required for endocavital studies, and the examination should be witnessed by another health care professional. Note that the initials of the witness should be included as part of the film labeling.
- Transabdominal pelvic studies require distention of the urinary bladder. Since this can cause patient discomfort, every effort should be made to perform the exam quickly.
- Experiment with using different amounts of transducer pressure on the skin surface. More often than not you can press the transducer harder than you realize and, in turn, improve image quality. Always make sure that the patient is comfortable.

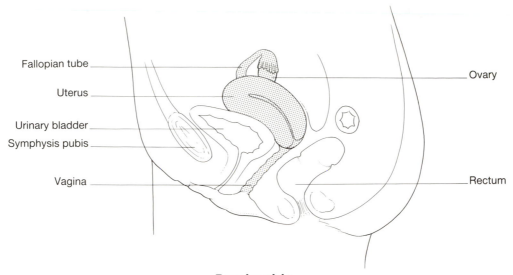

Female pelvis

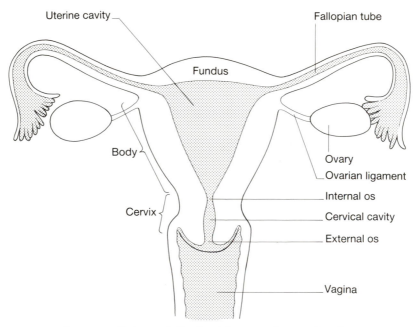

Anatomy of uterus, fallopian tubes, ovaries, and vagina

CHAPTER THIRTEEN
FEMALE PELVIS SCANNING
PROTOCOL

BETTY BATES TEMPKIN

LOCATION

- The urinary bladder is posterior to the symphysis pubis.

- The uterus, cervix, and vagina are posterior to the distended bladder and anterior to the rectum.

- The fundus of the uterus usually lies just to the right or left of midline.

- The cervix and vagina usually lie in the midline of the pelvic cavity.

- The ovaries are lateral to the uterus and lie against the pelvic side walls.

- The ureter and internal iliac vessels are posterior to the ovary.

ANATOMY

- The female pelvic cavity consists of the female reproductive organs, a portion of the ureters, the urinary bladder, musculature, and intestinal tract.

- The female reproductive system consists of the vagina, uterus, two fallopian tubes, and two ovaries.

- The adnexa consist of the ovaries, fallopian tubes, pelvic ligaments, and pelvic side walls.

- The vagina is a muscular, tubular structure that extends from the cervix of the uterus to the vulva.

- The uterus is a muscular, hollow organ. The size of the uterus is variable depending on patient parity and age. Postpubertal size is usually 7 to 8 cm long, 3 to 5 cm wide, and 3 to 5 cm thick.

- The uterus consists of three muscle layers:

  - Endometrium: The inner mucous layer.

  - Myometrium: The middle, smooth muscle, thickest layer.

  - Serous: The outer peritoneal layer.

- The uterus is pear-shaped; its rounded superior portion is the fundus and its inferior tapering portion is the cervix or neck. The middle portion of the uterus is referred to as its body.

- The uterus has a centrally located endometrial cavity. The cervical portion of the cavity where it meets the vagina is referred to as the external os and where it meets the uterine body is referred to as the internal os.

- The uterine cavity is continuous with the centrally located vaginal canal.

- The fallopian tubes arise from the uterus and course within the broad ligament for about 10 cm (4 in) toward the ovaries.

- The ovaries are oval-shaped organs that lie within the ovarian fossae against the pelvic sidewalls. The size of the ovaries is variable and depends on age. Postpubertal size is approximately 2 cm long, 2 cm wide, and 3 cm to 4 cm thick.

- The two ureters are long, narrow tubular structures that extend from the hilum of each kidney to the urinary bladder. The ureters are less than 1.4 in wide and 10 to 12 in long. The ureters decrease in diameter as they course to the bladder.

- The urinary bladder is a symmetrical, hollow, muscular organ. Bladder shape is variable depending on distention. The bladder can hold as much as 16 to 18 ounces of urine. The normal distended urinary bladder wall measures 1 cm or less.

- Pelvic side wall musculature includes:
  - Obturator internus muscle.
  - Iliopsoas muscle.
  - Piriformis muscle.
  - Pubococcygeal sling muscle.

PHYSIOLOGY

- The function of the uterus, vagina, and ovaries is reproduction.

- The function of the ureters is to carry urine from the hilum of each kidney to the urinary bladder.

- The function of the urinary bladder is to store urine until the urge to void is felt.

SONOGRAPHIC APPEARANCE

- The uterine myometrium is midgray or medium-level echoes with even texture. The contour of the normal myometrium should appear smooth. Occasionally round, anechoic venous structures may be seen along the uterine periphery.

- The endometrial cavity is a thin echogenic line that varies in intensity and thickness depending on the menstrual phase and patient age.

- The vaginal walls are midgray or medium-level echoes with even texture that is equal to the normal uterus. The vaginal canal is echogenic.

- The ovaries are midgray or medium-level echoes with even texture that is equal to or more echogenic than the normal uterus. Uterine follicles are seen as round or oval anechoic structures along the ovarian periphery.

- The fallopian tubes are not normally seen.

- The ureters are not normally seen.

- The urinary bladder cavity is not seen if it is collapsed; otherwise it appears anechoic. The bladder wall appears as a smooth, thin echogenic line. Distended bladder shape is variable but transversely it may appear somewhat squared.

- The pelvic side wall musculature is mid-gray or medium-level echoes with even texture that is less echogenic than the normal uterus and ovaries.
- The cul-de-sac or pouch of Douglas is a recessed portion of the peritoneum posterior to the uterus that is seen when it contains fluid or blood. It is normal to see a small amount of anechoic free fluid between the echogenic walls of the cul-de-sac and the myometrium of the uterus.

NORMAL VARIANTS

- Retroverted uterus:
  - The entire uterus is tilted posteriorly.
  - Sonographic appearance is the same as that of the normal uterus.
- Retroflexed uterus:
  - Only the uterine fundus and body are tilted posteriorly.
  - Sonographic appearance is the same as that of the normal uterus.
- Didelphia uterus:
  - Developmental variant causing two uterine bodies, two cervices, and two vaginas.
  - Sonographic appearance is the same as that of the normal uterus, cervix, and vagina.
- Bicornuate uterus:
  - Developmental variant causing two uterine bodies (divided) or two uterine horns (septated) with one vagina and one or two cervices.
  - Sonographic appearance is the same as that of the normal uterus, cervix, and vagina.

PATIENT PREP

- Full urinary bladder.
- 32 to 40 ounces of clear fluid should be ingested one hour before the exam and finished within a 15 to 20 minute time period.
- If for any reason the patient cannot have fluids, sterile water can be used to fill the bladder through a Foley catheter.

NOTE: The fully distended urinary bladder displaces the bowel and brings the pelvic organs into view. Note that an over-filled bladder can actually push the pelvic contents out of view. If so, have the patient partially void.

NOTE: Normal bowel can mimic pathology. To distinguish between the two, the patient can be given a water enema that will clarify the bowel.

PATIENT POSITION

- Supine.

TRANSDUCER

- **3.0 MHz** or **3.5 MHz**.
- 5.0 MHz for thin patients.

BREATHING TECHNIQUE

- Normal respiration.

FEMALE PELVIS SURVEY

NOTE: Prior to the examination a patient history should be taken to include the date of the first day of the patient's last period, parity, gravidity (pregnancy test results if available), symptoms, pelvic exam results, and history of pelvic surgery. Most sonography departments have standard forms where this information is recorded.

NOTE: Survey of the female pelvis begins with longitudinal and transverse surveys of the uterus and pelvic cavity followed by longitudinal and transverse surveys of the ovaries.

UTERUS AND PELVIC CAVITY SURVEY

LONGITUDINAL SURVEY

Sagittal Plane/Anterior Approach

● BEGIN WITH THE TRANSDUCER PERPENDICULAR, AT THE MIDLINE OF THE BODY, JUST SUPERIOR TO THE SYMPHYSIS PUBIS. IN MOST CASES THE VAGINA AND CERVIX WILL BE VISUALIZED HERE AND POSSIBLY THE BODY AND FUNDUS OF THE UTERUS DEPENDING ON THEIR LIE. IF THE VAGINA IS NOT SEEN, ANGLE THE TRANSDUCER INFERIORLY AND ROTATE THE TRANSDUCER VARYING DEGREES (TO OBLIQUE THE SCANNING PLANE ACCORDING TO THE LIE OF THE VAGINA) TO VISUALIZE THE VAGINA AND ITS LONG AXIS.

NOTE THE BLADDER ANTERIORLY.

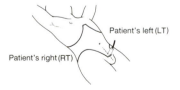

● ONCE THE LONG AXIS OF THE VAGINA IS LOCATED, ANGLE THE TRANSDUCER INFERIORLY TO SCAN THROUGH THE VAGINA UNTIL YOU ARE BEYOND IT.

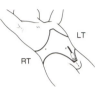

● RETURN TO THE MIDLINE JUST SUPERIOR TO THE SYMPHYSIS PUBIS. WITH THE TRANSDUCER PERPENDICULAR, LOCATE THE LONG AXIS OF THE UTERUS. IT MAY BE NECESSARY TO ROTATE THE TRANSDUCER VARYING DEGREES (TO OBLIQUE THE SCANNING PLANE ACCORDING TO UTERINE LIE) TO VISUALIZE THE LONG AXIS OF THE UTERUS.

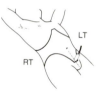

● ONCE THE LONG AXIS OF THE UTERUS IS LOCATED, SLOWLY MOVE THE TRANSDUCER TOWARD THE PATIENT'S RIGHT, SCANNING LATERALLY THROUGH THE UTERUS AND VAGINA UNTIL YOU ARE JUST BEYOND THEM.

NOTE THE BLADDER ANTERIORLY.

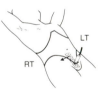

- CONTINUE TO SCAN RIGHT LATERAL THROUGH THE PELVIC SIDE WALL UNTIL YOU ARE BEYOND IT.

    NOTE THE BLADDER ANTERIORLY AND THE LOCATION OF THE RIGHT OVARY.

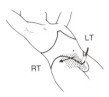

- RETURN TO MIDLINE, JUST SUPERIOR TO THE SYMPHYSIS PUBIS, AND LOCATE THE LONG AXIS OF THE UTERUS.

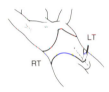

- ONCE THE LONG AXIS IS LOCATED, SLOWLY MOVE THE TRANSDUCER TOWARD THE PATIENT'S LEFT, SCANNING LATERALLY THROUGH THE UTERUS AND VAGINA UNTIL YOU ARE JUST BEYOND THEM.

    NOTE THE BLADDER ANTERIORLY.

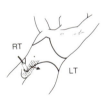

- CONTINUE TO SCAN LEFT LATERAL THROUGH THE PELVIC SIDE WALL UNTIL YOU ARE BEYOND IT.

NOTE THE BLADDER ANTERIORLY AND THE LOCATION OF THE LEFT OVARY.

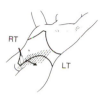

TRANSVERSE SURVEY

Transverse Plane/Anterior Approach

- BEGIN WITH THE TRANSDUCER ANGLED INFERIORLY, AT THE MIDLINE OF THE BODY, JUST SUPERIOR TO THE SYMPHYSIS PUBIS.

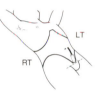

- ANGLE THE TRANSDUCER INFERIORLY ENOUGH THAT YOU ARE OUT OF THE PELVIS. *SLOWLY* ANGLE THE TRANSDUCER BACK INTO THE PELVIS, LOOKING FIRST FOR THE VAGINA.

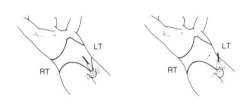

    NOTE THE BLADDER ANTERIORLY, RECTUM POSTERIORLY, AND THE SIDEWALLS.

NOTE: The normal traversed vagina, cervix, uterus body, and fundus appear as smooth, oval, organ textures with echogenic to hypoechoic centers. They gradually increase in size from the vagina to uterine fundus. Note that these structures lie between the distended anterior bladder and posterior bowel.

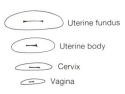

Uterine fundus

Uterine body

Cervix

Vagina

● WITH THE TRANSDUCER BECOMING PERPENDICULAR, SCAN SUPERIORLY THROUGH THE VAGINA AND ONTO THE CERVIX.

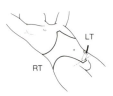

NOTE THE BLADDER ANTERIORLY, AREA OF THE CUL-DE-SAC POSTERIORLY, AND THE SIDE WALLS.
● SCANNING PERPENDICULAR AND SUPERIORLY THROUGH THE CERVIX, MOVE ONTO THE BODY OF THE UTERUS.

NOTE THE BLADDER ANTERIORLY, THE SIDE WALLS, AND THE LOCATION OF THE OVARIES.

● CONTINUE SCANNING SUPERIORLY THROUGH THE BODY OF THE UTERUS AND ONTO THE FUNDUS. SCAN SUPERIORLY THROUGH THE FUNDUS AND SUPERIOR BLADDER WALLS TO THE LEVEL OF THE UMBILICUS.

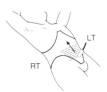

NOTE THE BLADDER ANTERIORLY, THE SIDE WALLS, AND THE LOCATION OF THE OVARIES. AS YOU SCAN BEYOND THE BLADDER, ADJUST TECHNIQUE ACCORDING TO BOWEL APPEARANCE.

OVARIES SURVEY

NOTE: The location of the ovaries is variable. They are generally lateral to the body or fundus of the uterus but may be found tucked in close to the side of the uterus. Other locations include posterior or superior to the uterus. If the ovaries are not identified during the following surveys, every effort must be made to locate them, including endovaginal sonography.

Right Ovary Survey

LONGITUDINAL SURVEY

Sagittal Plane/Anterior Approach

● BEGIN WITH THE TRANSDUCER PER-
PENDICULAR, AT THE MIDLINE OF THE
BODY, JUST SUPERIOR TO THE SYMPHY-
SIS PUBIS. RECALL THE LOCATION OF
THE RIGHT OVARY FROM THE PELVIC
CAVITY SURVEY.

● LOCATE THE LONG AXIS OF THE UTER-
US, THEN SLOWLY MOVE THE TRANS-
DUCER RIGHT LATERAL UNTIL THE RIGHT
OVARY IS LOCATED. LOOK FOR THE LON-
GITUDINAL INTERNAL ILIAC VESSELS IM-
MEDIATELY POSTERIOR TO THE OVARY.
IT MAY BE NECESSARY TO SLIGHTLY RO-
TATE THE TRANSDUCER TO RESOLVE
THE LIE OF THE OVARY.

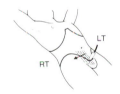

NOTE: If the ovary cannot be seen because of overlying bowel, angle the transducer right lateral toward the right ovary
from the midline of the pelvic cavity or
just to the left of the midline.

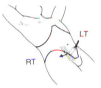

● ONCE THE OVARY IS LOCATED, MOVE
OR ANGLE THE TRANSDUCER RIGHT LAT-
ERAL, SCANNING THROUGH AND BEYOND
THE LATERAL MARGIN OF THE OVARY.

● MOVE BACK ONTO THE OVARY AND
MOVE OR ANGLE THE TRANSDUCER TO-
WARD THE MIDLINE OF THE PELVIC CAV-
ITY, SCANNING THROUGH AND BEYOND
THE MEDIAL MARGIN OF THE OVARY.

● MOVE BACK ONTO THE RIGHT OVARY.

TRANSVERSE SURVEY

Transverse Plane/Anterior Approach

● STILL VIEWING THE LONGITUDINAL RIGHT OVARY IN THE SAGITTAL PLANE, ROTATE THE TRANSDUCER 90 DEGREES INTO THE TRANSVERSE SCANNING PLANE TO TRAVERSE THE RIGHT OVARY.

NOTE THE TRAVERSED INTERNAL ILIAC VESSELS POSTERIOR TO THE OVARY.

● MOVE OR ANGLE THE TRANSDUCER SUPERIORLY, SCANNING THROUGH AND BEYOND THE SUPERIOR MARGIN OF THE OVARY.

● MOVE BACK ONTO THE OVARY AND MOVE OR ANGLE THE TRANSDUCER INFERIORLY, SCANNING THROUGH AND BEYOND THE INFERIOR MARGIN OF THE OVARY.

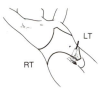

Left Ovary Survey

USE THE SAME SURVEY SCANNING METHODS AS THOSE FOR THE RIGHT OVARY.

REQUIRED PICTURES

Pelvic Cavity and Uterus

LONGITUDINAL IMAGES

Sagittal Plane/Anterior Approach

NOTE: Longitudinal images begin with survey images of the pelvic cavity to be followed by a long axis image of the uterus.

1. LONGITUDINAL IMAGE OF THE MIDLINE OF THE PELVIC CAVITY JUST SUPERIOR TO THE SYMPHYSIS PUBIS.

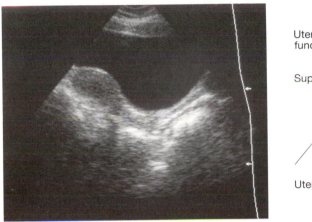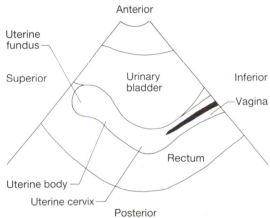

LABELED: PELVIS SAG ML

2. LONGITUDINAL IMAGE OF THE RIGHT ADNEXA THAT MAY INCLUDE PART OF THE UTERUS DEPENDING ON ITS LIE.

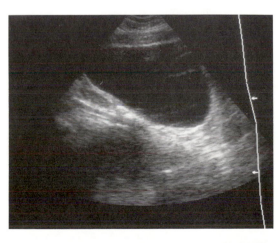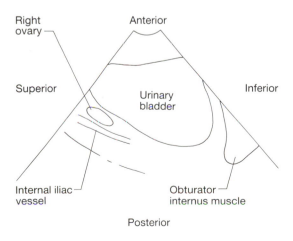

LABELED: PELVIS SAG R1

3. LONGITUDINAL IMAGE TO INCLUDE THE RIGHT LATERAL WALL OF THE BLADDER AND PELVIC SIDE WALL.

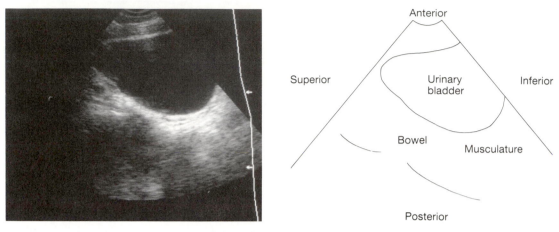

LABELED: PELVIS SAG R2

4. LONGITUDINAL IMAGE OF THE LEFT ADNEXA THAT MAY INCLUDE PART OF THE UTERUS DEPENDING ON ITS LIE.

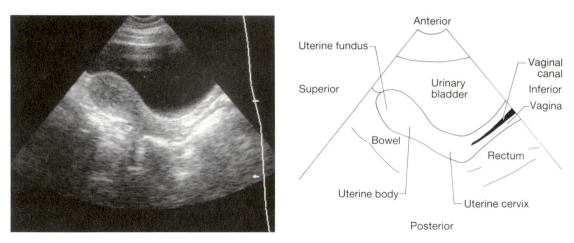

LABELED: PELVIS SAG L1

5. LONGITUDINAL IMAGE TO INCLUDE THE LEFT LATERAL WALL OF THE BLADDER AND PELVIC SIDE WALL.

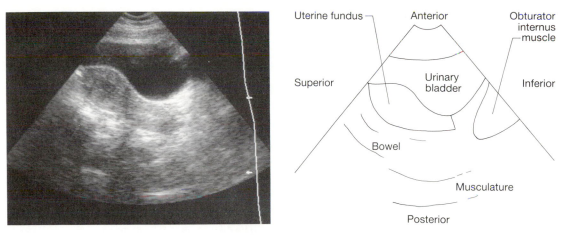

LABELED: PELVIS SAG L2

6. LONG AXIS IMAGE OF THE UTERUS TO INCLUDE AS MUCH ENDOMETRIAL CAVITY AS POSSIBLE WITH *SUPERIOR TO INFERIOR AND ANTERIOR TO POSTERIOR MEASUREMENT.*

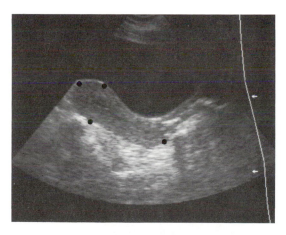

LABELED: UT SAG LONG AXIS

7. SAME IMAGE AS NUMBER 6 WITHOUT CALIPERS.

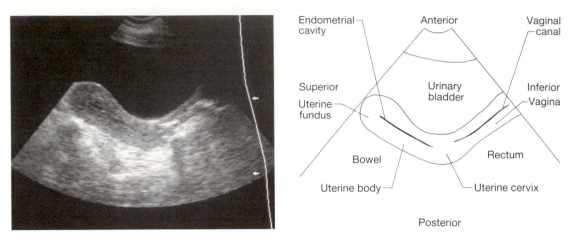

LABELED: UT SAG LONG AXIS

NOTE: It may be necessary to take a separate image of the endometrial cavity. If so, label: **UT SAG**

TRANSVERSE IMAGES

Transverse Plane/Anterior Approach

8. TRANSVERSE IMAGE OF THE VAGINA.

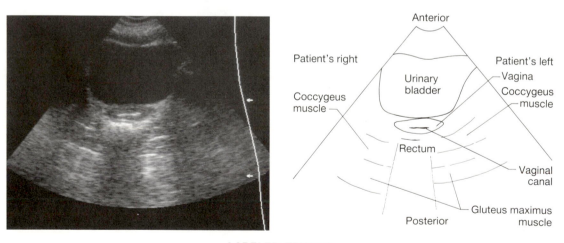

LABELED: TRV VAG

9. TRANSVERSE IMAGE OF THE CERVIX.

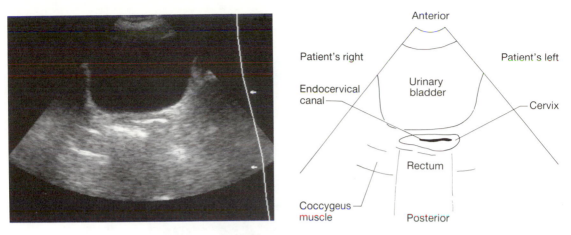

LABELED: TRV CERX

10. TRANSVERSE IMAGE OF THE UTERUS BODY.

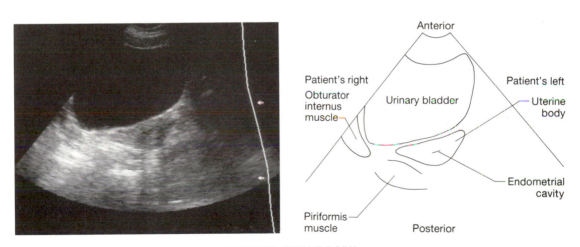

LABELED: TRV UT BODY

11. TRANSVERSE IMAGE OF THE UTERUS FUNDUS WITH *RIGHT TO LEFT MEASUREMENT*.

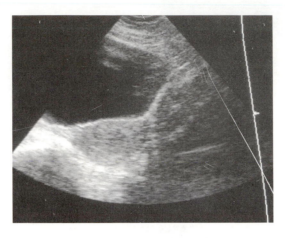

LABELED: TRV UT FUNDUS

12. SAME IMAGE AS NUMBER 11 WITHOUT CALIPERS.

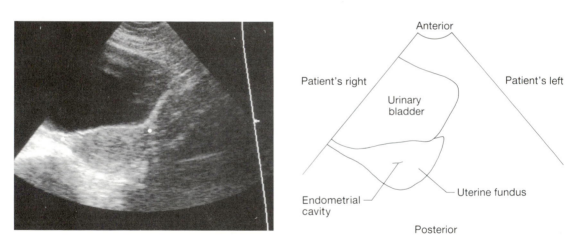

LABELED: TRV UT FUNDUS

Right Ovary

NOTE: Due to the variability of the location and lie of the ovaries the long axis can lie in any scanning plane. The following images reflect the long axis in the sagittal plane.

LONGITUDINAL IMAGE

Sagittal Plane/Anterior Approach

13. LONG AXIS IMAGE OF THE RIGHT OVARY WITH *SUPERIOR TO INFERIOR AND ANTERIOR TO POSTERIOR MEASUREMENT*.

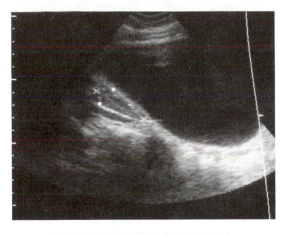

LABELED: RT OV SAG LONG AXIS

NOTE: If this image of the ovary was angled from midline then the image is obliqued and must be labeled: **RT OV SAG OBL LONG AXIS**

14. SAME IMAGE AS NUMBER 13 WITHOUT CALIPERS.

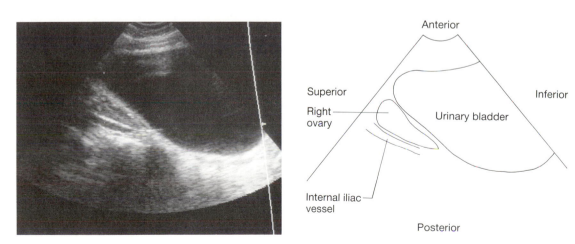

LABELED: RT OV SAG LONG AXIS

TRANSVERSE IMAGE

Transverse Plane/Anterior Approach

15. TRANSVERSE IMAGE OF THE RIGHT OVARY WITH *RIGHT TO LEFT MEAS-UREMENT*.

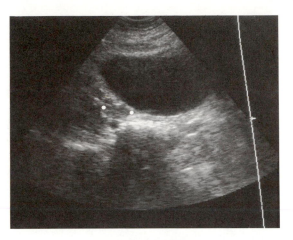

LABELED: RT OV TRV

NOTE: If this is an oblique image then label: **RT OV TRV OBL**

16. SAME IMAGE AS NUMBER 15 WITHOUT CALIPERS.

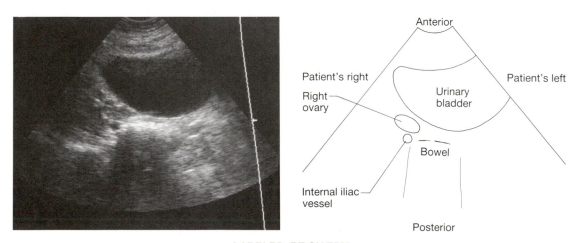

LABELED: RT OV TRV

Left Ovary

LONGITUDINAL IMAGE

Sagittal Plane/Anterior Approach

17. LONG AXIS IMAGE OF THE LEFT OVARY WITH *SUPERIOR TO INFERIOR AND ANTERIOR TO POSTERIOR MEASUREMENT.*

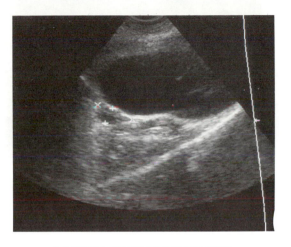

LABELED: LT OV SAG LONG AXIS

NOTE: If this is an oblique image then label: **LT OV SAG OBL LONG AXIS**

18. SAME IMAGE AS NUMBER 17 WITHOUT CALIPERS.

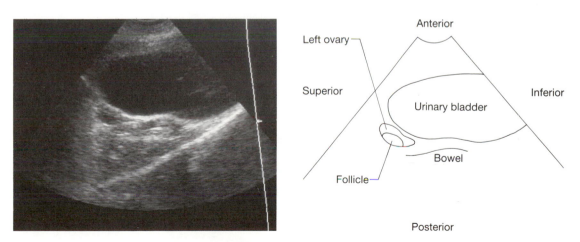

LABELED: LT OV SAG LONG AXIS

TRANSVERSE IMAGE

Transverse Plane/Anterior Approach

19. TRANSVERSE IMAGE OF THE LEFT OVARY WITH *RIGHT TO LEFT MEAS-UREMENT*.

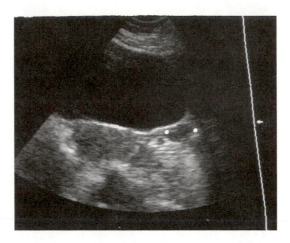

LABELED: LT OV TRV

NOTE: If this is an obliqued image then label: **LT OV OBL TRV**

20. SAME IMAGE AS NUMBER 19 WITHOUT CALIPERS.

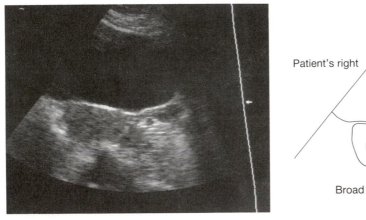

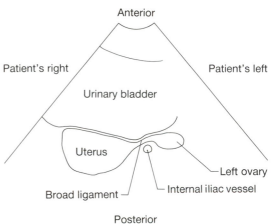

LABELED: LT OV TRV

ENDOVAGINAL SONOGRAPHY

BETTY BATES TEMPKIN and KRISTIN DYKSTRA-DOWNEY

NOTE: In most cases endovaginal sonography is used in conjunction with transabdominal sonography when pelvic contents require further evaluation. If the transabdominal scan provides the diagnosis then the endovaginal scan is not necessary.

PATIENT PREP

- Explain the examination to the patient. Inform the patient that the exam is virtually painless, that the inserted transducer feels like a tampon, and the exam is necessary for an accurate diagnosis. Verbal or written consent is required, and the exam should be witnessed by a female health care professional. Note that the initials of the witness should be included as part of the film labeling.

- Empty urinary bladder.

- The transducer may be inserted by the patient, sonographer, or physician.

PATIENT POSITION

- Transducer design determines patient position so ideally having a gynecological examining table and the ability to put the patient in lithotomy position is optimal.

- Another option is positioning the patient at the end of the examining table or stretcher with the hips elevated by a pillow or foam cushion.

TRANSDUCER

- **5 MHz to 7.5 MHz.**

- Apply gel to the end of the transducer, then cover it with a condom, finger of a rubber glove, or sheath. Make sure there are no air bubbles at the tip, then apply additional gel to the outside of the condom before insertion. If infertility is a consideration, then water or nonspermicidal gel may be used.

ORIENTATION

NOTE: Endovaginal scanning is technically organ-oriented, but the following scanning planes are currently being used for image interpretation.

- Sagittal (longitudinal) and coronal (transverse) views of the pelvic organs are obtained.

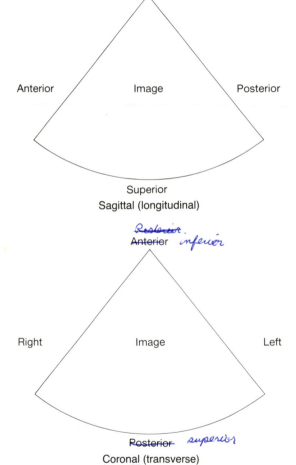

Inferior

Anterior   Image   Posterior

Superior
Sagittal (longitudinal)

Posterior
Anterior *inferior*

Right   Image   Left

Posterior *superior*
Coronal (transverse)

SURVEY

NOTE: The inserted transducer must be slightly angled in different directions to visualize the uterus and adnexa.

Uterus Survey

LONGITUDINAL SURVEY

Sagittal Plane/Vaginal Approach

- BEGIN BY SLOWLY LOWERING THE TRANSDUCER HANDLE TOWARD THE FLOOR TO VIEW THE FUNDUS OF THE UTERUS. SLIGHTLY MOVE THE TRANSDUCER TO THE RIGHT AND LEFT TO EVALUATE THE LATERAL MARGINS.
  NOTE THE ENDOMETRIAL CAVITY. IF THE BLADDER CONTAINS ANY URINE, NOTE IT ANTERIORLY OR ON THE LEFT SIDE OF THE IMAGING SCREEN.
- WITHDRAW THE TRANSDUCER SLIGHTLY, AND SLOWLY LIFT THE HANDLE TOWARD THE CEILING TO VIEW THE BODY OF THE UTERUS, CERVIX, AND CUL-DE-SAC. MOVE THE TRANSDUCER TO THE RIGHT AND LEFT TO EVALUATE THE LATERAL MARGINS.
  NOTE THE ENDOMETRIAL CAVITY.

NOTE: Move the transducer in opposite directions for a retroverted uterus, or it may be helpful to invert the probe 180 degrees.

TRANSVERSE SURVEY

Coronal Plane/Vaginal Approach

- ROTATE THE TRANSDUCER 90 DEGREES INTO THE CORONAL PLANE.
- BEGIN BY SLOWLY LOWERING THE TRANSDUCER HANDLE TOWARD THE FLOOR TO EVALUATE THE ANTERIOR MARGINS OF THE FUNDUS.
- WITHDRAW THE TRANSDUCER SLIGHTLY AND LIFT THE HANDLE TOWARD THE CEILING TO EVALUATE THE POSTERIOR MARGINS OF THE UTERUS, CERVIX, AND CUL-DE-SAC.

Ovaries Survey

RIGHT OVARY

Transverse Survey

Coronal Plane/Vaginal Approach

● BEGIN BY PUTTING THE TRANSDUCER IN A RIGHT OBLIQUE POSITION. THIS IS DONE BY MOVING THE TRANSDUCER HANDLE AGAINST THE PATIENT'S LEFT THIGH, WHICH ANGLES THE BEAM TOWARD THE RIGHT ADNEXA.

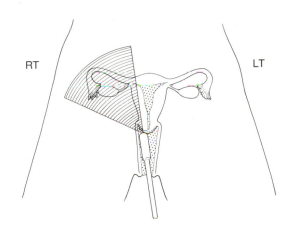

● FIND THE OVARY BY SLIGHTLY MOVING THE TRANSDUCER HANDLE UP AND DOWN.

  NOTE THE ADJACENT ILIAC VESSELS.
● ONCE THE OVARY IS LOCATED, MOVE THE TRANSDUCER HANDLE UP AND DOWN TO SCAN THROUGH THE ANTERIOR AND POSTERIOR MARGINS.

Longitudinal Survey

Sagittal Plane/Vaginal Approach

● STILL VIEWING THE OVARY IN THE CORONAL PLANE, ROTATE THE TRANSDUCER 90 DEGREES INTO THE SAGITTAL PLANE.
● BEGIN BY VERY SLIGHTLY MOVING THE TRANSDUCER HANDLE TO THE RIGHT AND LEFT TO SCAN THROUGH THE LATERAL AND MEDIAL MARGINS.

  NOTE THE ADJACENT ILIAC VESSELS.

LEFT OVARY

● BEGIN BY PUTTING THE TRANSDUCER IN A LEFT OBLIQUE POSITION. THIS IS DONE BY MOVING THE TRANSDUCER HANDLE AGAINST THE PATIENT'S RIGHT THIGH. FOLLOW THE SAME SURVEY METHODS AS FOR THE RIGHT OVARY FOR TRANSVERSE AND LONGITUDINAL SURVEYS.

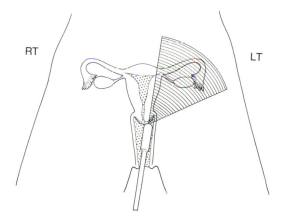

REQUIRED PICTURES*

Uterus

LONGITUDINAL IMAGES

Sagittal Plane/Vaginal Approach

1. LONGITUDINAL MIDLINE IMAGE THAT MAY INCLUDE THE LONG AXIS OF THE UTERUS. LONG AXIS TO INCLUDE *SUPERIOR TO INFERIOR AND ANTERIOR TO POSTERIOR MEASUREMENTS.*

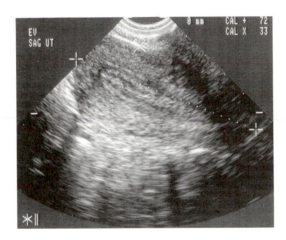

LABELED: EV SAG ML OR EV SAG ML UT LONG AXIS
("EV" INDICATES ENDOVAGINAL)

NOTE: If the long axis is not imaged at midline it should be taken here and labeled: **EV SAG UT LONG AXIS**

2. SAME IMAGE AS NUMBER 1 WITHOUT CALIPERS.

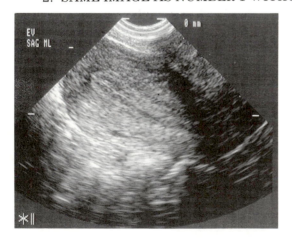
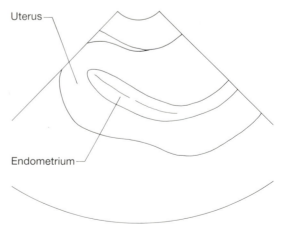

LABELED: EV SAG ML UT LONG AXIS

*Images in this section are by courtesy of Thomas Jefferson University, Philadelphia, Pennsylvania.

NOTE: Because of the limited field of view some of the uterus may not be visible on the long axis. If so, take these additional images:

> 3. LONGITUDINAL IMAGE OF THE UTERUS FUNDUS TO INCLUDE THE EN-DOMETRIAL CAVITY.

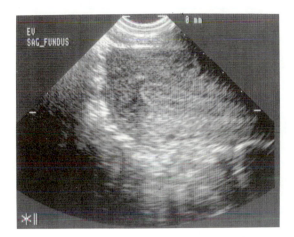 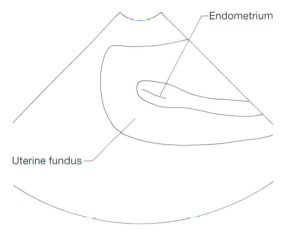

LABELED: EV SAG FUNDUS

> 4. LONGITUDINAL IMAGE OF THE UTERUS BODY AND CERVIX TO INCLUDE THE ENDOMETRIAL CAVITY.

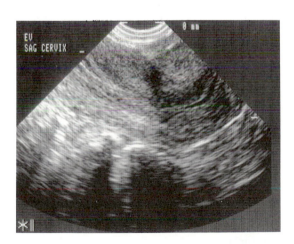 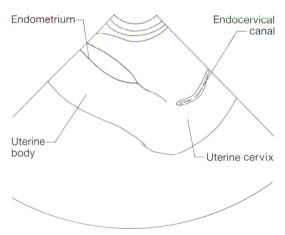

LABELED: EV SAG BODY CERX

TRANSVERSE IMAGES

Coronal Plane/Vaginal Approach

5. TRANSVERSE IMAGE OF THE UTERUS FUNDUS WITH *RIGHT TO LEFT MEASUREMENT*.

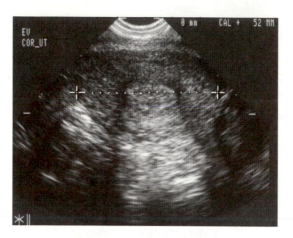

LABELED: EV COR FUNDUS

6. SAME IMAGE AS NUMBER 5 WITHOUT CALIPERS.

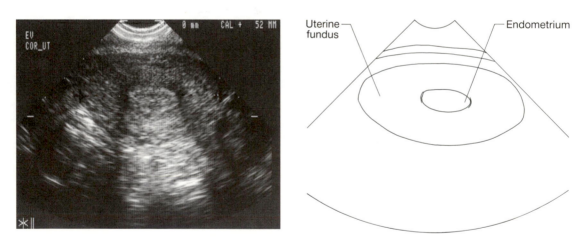

LABELED: EV COR FUNDUS

7. TRANSVERSE IMAGE OF THE UTERUS BODY.

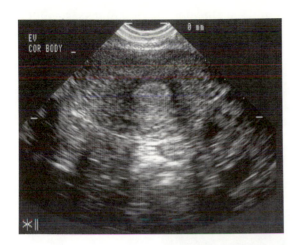
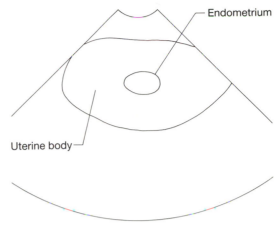

Endometrium

Uterine body

LABELED: EV COR BODY

8. TRANSVERSE IMAGE OF THE CERVIX.

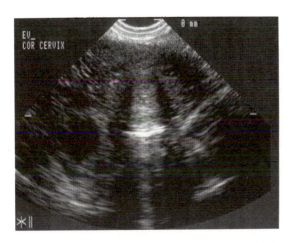
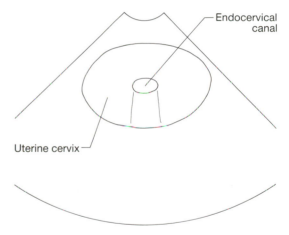

Endocervical canal

Uterine cervix

LABELED: EV COR CERX

Right Ovary

NOTE: Due to the variability of the location and lie of the ovaries the long axis can lie in any scanning plane. The following images reflect the long axis in the sagittal plane.

TRANSVERSE IMAGE

Coronal Plane/Vaginal Approach

9. TRANSVERSE IMAGE OF THE RIGHT OVARY WITH *RIGHT TO LEFT MEASUREMENT*.

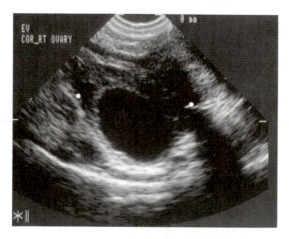

LABELED: EV COR RT OV

10. SAME IMAGE AS NUMBER 9 WITHOUT CALIPERS.

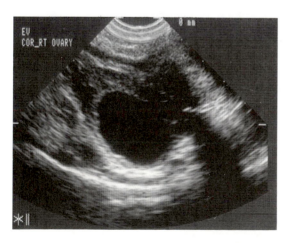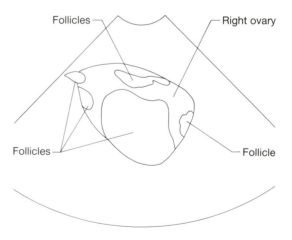

LABELED: EV COR RT OV

LONGITUDINAL IMAGE

Sagittal Plane/Vaginal Approach

11. LONG AXIS IMAGE OF THE RIGHT OVARY WITH *SUPERIOR TO INFERIOR AND ANTERIOR TO POSTERIOR MEASUREMENTS*.

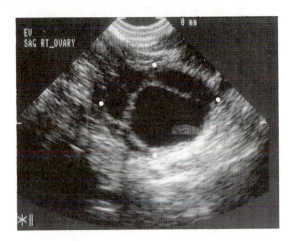

LABELED: EV SAG RT OV LONG AXIS

12. SAME IMAGE AS NUMBER 11 WITHOUT CALIPERS.

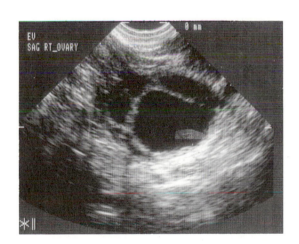 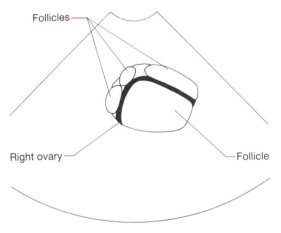

LABELED: EV SAG RT OV LONG AXIS

Left Ovary

TRANSVERSE IMAGE

Coronal Plane/Vaginal Approach

13. TRANSVERSE IMAGE OF THE LEFT OVARY WITH *RIGHT TO LEFT MEASUREMENT*.

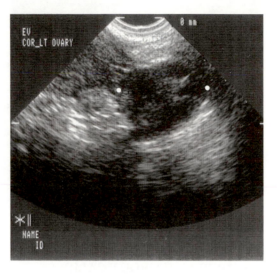

LABELED: EV COR LT OV

14. SAME IMAGE AS NUMBER 13 WITHOUT CALIPERS.

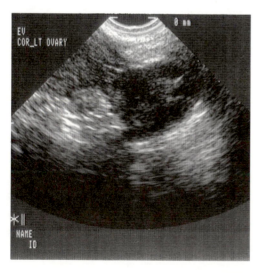

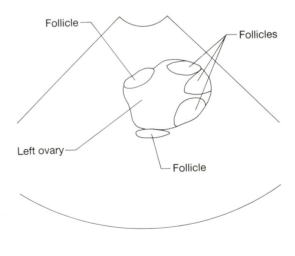

LABELED: EV COR LT OV

LONGITUDINAL IMAGE

Sagittal Plane/Vaginal Approach

15. LONG AXIS IMAGE OF THE LEFT OVARY WITH *SUPERIOR TO INFERIOR AND ANTERIOR TO POSTERIOR MEASUREMENTS.*

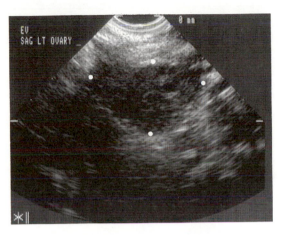

LABELED: EV SAG LT OV LONG AXIS

16. SAME IMAGE AS NUMBER 15 WITHOUT CALIPERS.

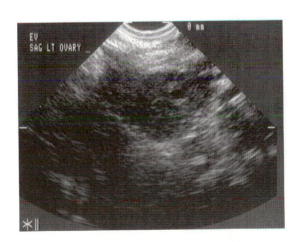 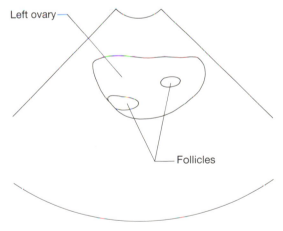

LABELED: EV SAG LT OV LONG AXIS

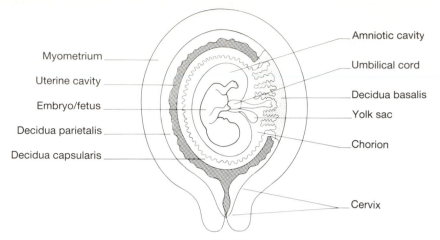

Myometrium

Uterine cavity

Embryo/fetus

Decidua parietalis

Decidua capsularis

Amniotic cavity

Umbilical cord

Decidua basalis

Yolk sac

Chorion

Cervix

First trimester

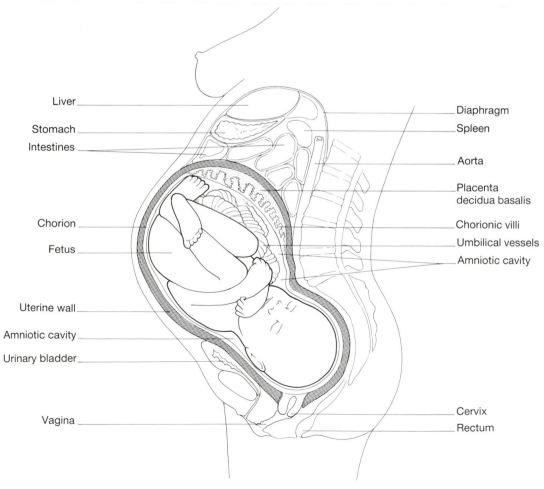

Liver

Stomach

Intestines

Chorion

Fetus

Uterine wall

Amniotic cavity

Urinary bladder

Vagina

Diaphragm

Spleen

Aorta

Placenta
decidua basalis

Chorionic villi

Umbilical vessels

Amniotic cavity

Cervix

Rectum

Third trimester

CHAPTER FOURTEEN
OBSTETRICAL SCANNING
PROTOCOL

ANATOMY

MATERNAL ANATOMY

- Maternal pelvic cavity includes the vagina, uterus, two ovaries, two fallopian tubes, a portion of the ureters, the urinary bladder, musculature, and intestinal tract. Refer to Chapter 13 for anatomical specifics.

FIRST TRIMESTER ANATOMY AND SONOGRAPHIC APPEARANCE

- Gestational sac. Represents the anechoic fluid-filled chorionic cavity surrounded by the echogenic trophoblast. Normal locations include middle and fundal portions of the uterus. Early in the trimester, the echogenic embryo and yolk sac can be visualized within the gestational sac. The yolk sac disappears between the 10th and 12th weeks of the trimester.

- Fetal cardiac activity may be visible as early as 4 weeks transvaginally and 6 weeks transabdominally. The fetal heart will appear small and pulsatile. The walls and contour appear echogenic, and the chambers are anechoic.

- Later in the trimester the echogenic cra-

nium, abdomen, and fetal limbs can be visualized.

- During the final stages of the trimester, the amnion and chorion fuse, forming the sonolucent fluid-filled amniotic cavity.

SECOND AND THIRD TRIMESTER ANATOMY AND SONOGRAPHIC APPEARANCE

- The parenchyma of the placenta appears midgray to low gray with relatively even texture. As the gestation advances, the parenchyma is interrupted by echogenic calcium deposits and/or sonolucent vessels. The fetal and maternal placental surfaces appear echogenic. The position of the placenta is variable within the uterus and may change as the uterus expands to accommodate the growing fetus.

- The fetal skeleton and extremities appear echogenic.

- The normal fetal spine will appear as an echogenic closed circle when traversed. Longitudinally it appears as two echogenic, curvilinear lines that widen at the skull and narrow at the sacrum.

- The fetal diaphragm appears as an echogenic, thin, curvilinear line that is easiest to visualize when you scan along the longitudinal axis of the fetus.

- The parenchyma of the fetal organs appears as midgray echo textures.

- The fetal urinary bladder, gallbladder, and stomach appear anechoic if fluid-filled surrounded by echogenic walls. If collapsed they are not visualized. The fetal intestine appears anechoic if fluid-filled, otherwise echogenic.

- The umbilical cord and other fetal vessels appear as echogenic walls with anechoic lumina.

- The walls and contour of the heart appear echogenic. The chambers of the heart appear anechoic.

- The contour of the normal fetal head is smooth, echogenic, and elliptical in shape.

- Intracranial anatomy from superior to inferior:

  – Interhemispheric fissure:

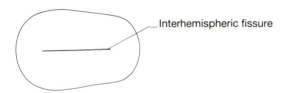

Interhemispheric fissure

A single, linear, echogenic structure visualized at the midline of the brain.

  – Lateral ventricles:

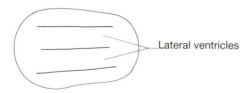

Lateral ventricles

The lateral walls appear as echogenic, linear structures lying the same distance from the interhemispheric fissure. The medial walls

when visualized appear echogenic. The chambers of the ventricles appear anechoic. Ventricular width is normal up to 10 mm.

The echogenic choroid plexus can be seen within the ventricular chambers.

– Thalamus, third ventricle, cavum septi pellucidi, frontal and occipital horns of the lateral ventricles:

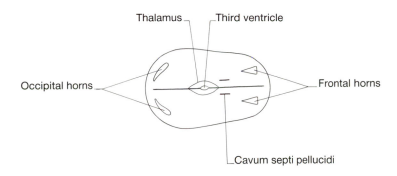

The thalamus is two large egg-shaped masses that lie on each side of the third ventricle. They appear midgray or as medium- to low-level echoes.

The third ventricle lies at the midline and appears as a small anechoic cavity with echogenic walls.

The cavum septi pellucidi lies at the midline and appears as an anechoic structure with echogenic, rectangular-shaped walls. It is located between the anterior border of the thalami and the frontal horns of the lateral ventricles.

The frontal horns of the lateral ventricles can be seen anteriorly and the occipital horns posteriorly.

The middle cerebral arteries may be seen pulsating within the lateral Sylvian fissures.

– Cerebral peduncles, basilar artery, and circle of Willis:

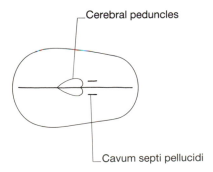

The cerebral peduncles are two heart-shaped masses that lie on each side of the midline. They appear similar in shape and texture to the thalami, but they are smaller and surrounded by thicker echoes. The parenchyma of the peduncles appears midgray or as medium- to low-level echoes.

The basilar artery can be seen pulsating at the midline between the anterior portions of the peduncles.

The circle of Willis can be seen pulsating at the midline anterior to the peduncles.

Base of the skull:

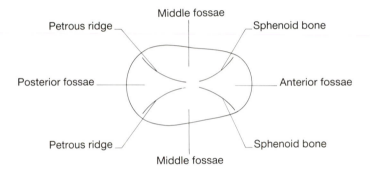

The anechoic anterior, middle, and posterior fossae are divided from each other by echogenic petrous ridges posteriorly and the echogenic sphenoid bones anteriorly.

Patient Prep

● Full urinary bladder.

● 32 to 40 ounces of clear fluid should be ingested 1 hour before the exam and finished within a 15- to 20-minute time period.

● If for any reason the patient cannot have fluids, sterile water can be used to fill the bladder through a Foley catheter.

NOTE: The fully distended urinary bladder displaces the bowel and brings the pelvic organs into view. Note that an overfilled bladder can actually push the pelvic contents out of view. If so, have the patient partially void.

ENDOVAGINAL PATIENT PREP

- See Chapter 13 for patient prep specifics.

PATIENT POSITION

- **Supine.**
- During the third trimester if the fetal head is in the lower uterine segment it may be helpful to elevate the patient's hips with a pillow or foam cushion.

ENDOVAGINAL PATIENT POSITION

- See Chapter 13 for patient position specifics.

TRANSDUCER

- **3.0** to **3.5 MHz.**
- 5.0 MHz for thin patients and third trimester fetal structures that may be close to the skin surface.

ENDOVAGINAL TRANSDUCER

- See Chapter 13 for transducer specifics.

OBSTETRICAL SURVEY

NOTE: Prior to the examination, a patient history should be taken to include the date of the first day of the patient's last period, gravidity, parity, and history of pelvic surgery. Most sonography departments have standard forms where this information is recorded.

NOTE: The obstetrical survey begins with longitudinal and transverse surveys of the uterus and adnexa to be followed by longitudinal and transverse surveys of the fetus.

Uterus and Adnexa Survey

Longitudinal Survey

Sagittal Plane/Anterior Approach

NOTE: While surveying the uterus and adnexa also verify **fetal life** and note if the pregnancy is **multiple**. Determine the fetal **lie and presentation**. Note the location of the **placenta**. Evaluate **amniotic fluid volume** subjectively; extremes are obvious.

NOTE: Fetal lie is determined by comparing the long axis of the fetus to the long axis of the uterus. Presentation refers to the fetal part closest to the cervix.

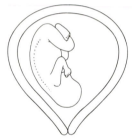

Longitudinal lie/cephalic presentation

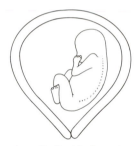

Longitudinal lie/breech presentation

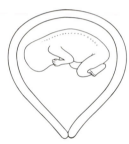

Transverse lie/head maternal right

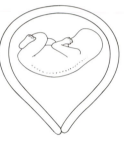

Transverse lie/head maternal left

● BEGIN WITH THE TRANSDUCER PERPENDICULAR, AT THE MIDLINE OF THE BODY, JUST SUPERIOR TO THE SYMPHYSIS PUBIS. IN MOST CASES THE VAGINA AND CERVIX WILL BE LOCATED HERE AND POSSIBLY THE BODY AND FUNDUS OF THE UTERUS, DEPENDING ON THEIR LIE AND THEIR SIZE ACCORDING TO THE TRIMESTER. IF THE VAGINA IS NOT SEEN, ANGLE THE TRANSDUCER INFERIORLY

AND ROTATE THE TRANSDUCER TO RE-SOLVE THE VAGINA AND ITS LONG AXIS.

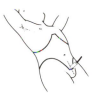

● ONCE THE VAGINA IS LOCATED, ANGLE THE TRANSDUCER INFERIORLY TO SCAN THROUGH THE VAGINA UNTIL YOU ARE BEYOND IT.

● RETURN TO THE MIDLINE JUST SUPE-RIOR TO THE SYMPHYSIS PUBIS.

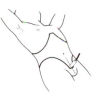

   EVALUATE THE CERVIX AND THE AREA OF THE CUL-DE-SAC POSTERI-ORLY. SLIGHTLY ROTATING THE TRANS-DUCER MAY HELP RESOLVE THE CERVIX.

● MOVE SUPERIORLY THROUGH THE CERVIX AND ALONG THE MIDLINE TO THE LEVEL OF THE UMBILICUS. EVALUATE WHATEVER PART OF THE UTERUS THAT MAY LIE HERE.

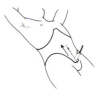

● RETURN TO THE MIDLINE JUST SUPE-RIOR TO THE SYMPHYSIS PUBIS. KEEP THE TRANSDUCER PERPENDICULAR AND SLOWLY MOVE THE TRANSDUCER TO-WARD THE PATIENT'S RIGHT SIDE, SCAN-NING THROUGH THE UTERUS AND THE ADNEXA UNTIL YOU ARE BEYOND IT.

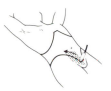

NOTE: As you scan laterally also move superiorly to evaluate the entire uterine fundus and its contents. Uterine lie is nor-mally variable and its size is dependent on the trimester.

● RETURN TO THE MIDLINE AND MOVE THE TRANSDUCER TOWARD THE PA-TIENT'S LEFT SIDE, SCANNING THROUGH THE UTERUS AND THE ADNEXA UNTIL YOU ARE BEYOND IT.

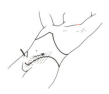

Transverse Survey

Transverse Plane/Anterior Approach

• BEGIN WITH THE TRANSDUCER AN-GLED INFERIORLY, AT THE MIDLINE, JUST SUPERIOR TO THE SYMPHYSIS PUBIS.

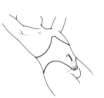

• ANGLE THE TRANSDUCER INFERIORLY ENOUGH THAT YOU ARE OUT OF THE PEL-VIS. *SLOWLY* ANGLE THE TRANSDUCER BACK INTO THE PELVIS LOOKING FIRST FOR THE VAGINA.

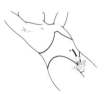

NOTE THE BLADDER ANTERIORLY, RECTUM POSTERIORLY, AND THE SIDE WALLS.
• WITH THE TRANSDUCER BECOMING PERPENDICULAR, SCAN SUPERIORLY THROUGH THE VAGINA AND ONTO THE CERVIX.

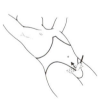

NOTE THE AREA OF THE CUL-DE-SAC POSTERIORLY AND THE SIDE WALLS.

• CONTINUE TO SCAN SUPERIORLY THROUGH THE CERVIX, BODY, AND FUN-DUS OF THE UTERUS. AS YOU MOVE SU-PERIORLY, ALSO EVALUATE THE AD-NEXA.

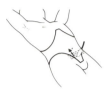

• SCAN SUPERIORLY THROUGH AND BE-YOND THE FUNDUS TO THE LEVEL OF THE UMBILICUS OR FURTHER ACCORDING TO UTERINE SIZE.

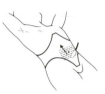

NOTE: As you scan superiorly also move laterally to completely evaluate the uterus and adnexa as the gestation progresses and the uterus becomes larger.

Fetal Survey

FIRST TRIMESTER SURVEY

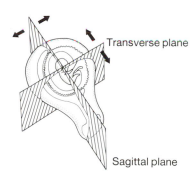

Transverse plane

Sagittal plane

Longitudinal Survey

Sagittal Plane/Anterior Approach

● BEGIN BY RESOLVING THE LONG AXIS OF THE UTERUS AND LOCATING THE GESTATIONAL SAC WITHIN.

● MOVE THE TRANSDUCER RIGHT LATERAL THROUGH AND BEYOND THE GESTATIONAL SAC THEN LEFT LATERAL THROUGH AND BEYOND THE SAC.

   NOTE AND EVALUATE ANY CONTENTS. VERY EARLY IN THE GESTATION THE SAC WILL NORMALLY APPEAR EMPTY. AS THE GESTATION PROGRESSES THE SMALL YOLK SAC, DEVELOPING AMNIOTIC SAC, DEVELOPING EMBRYO, DEVELOPING PLACENTA, AND UMBILICAL CORD CAN BE VISUALIZED.

● WHEN THE EMBRYO IS VISUALIZED, MAGNIFY THE FIELD OF VIEW AND LOOK FOR THE PULSATING HEART.

Transverse Survey

Transverse Plane/Anterior Approach

● STILL VIEWING THE GESTATIONAL SAC IN THE SAGITTAL PLANE ROTATE THE TRANSDUCER 90 DEGREES INTO THE TRANSVERSE PLANE.

● WITH THE TRANSDUCER PERPENDICULAR, BEGIN BY MOVING SUPERIORLY THROUGH AND BEYOND THE GESTATIONAL SAC THEN INFERIOR THROUGH AND BEYOND THE SAC. NOTE AND EVALUATE ANY CONTENTS.

SECOND AND THIRD TRIMESTER SURVEY

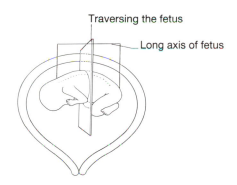

Traversing the fetus

Long axis of fetus

NOTE: Begin in the scanning plane where you visualized the long axis of the fetus during the survey of the uterus. Fetal position is variable, so the lie of the long axis may change. Change the scanning plane accordingly.

● LOCATE THE LONG AXIS OF THE FETUS. SLOWLY MOVE THROUGH THE FETUS NOTING THE FETAL HEART, LUNGS, AND DIAPHRAGM. ALSO EVALUATE THE ABDOMINOPELVIC CONTENTS INCLUDING THE KIDNEYS, LIVER, IVC, AND AORTA. THE GALLBLADDER, STOMACH, AND URINARY BLADDER CAN BE EXAMINED IF FLUID-FILLED. NOTE THE BOWEL.

NOTE: The examination is not complete until a significant amount of time has been given to visualize the fetal urinary bladder. Nonvisualization may be interpreted as nonfunctioning fetal kidneys.

• LOCATE THE LONG AXIS OF THE FETAL SPINE. ROTATING THE TRANSDUCER SLIGHTLY MAY AID VISUALIZATION. KEEP THE TRANSDUCER PERPENDICULAR AND SLOWLY MOVE ALONG THE SPINE THROUGH THE SACRAL END, THEN THROUGH THE SUPERIOR END TO THE SKULL. NOTE THAT THE SPINE NARROWS AT THE SACRUM AND WIDENS AT THE SKULL. ANY OTHER DEVIATIONS SEEN ALONG THE "DOUBLE LINE"–APPEARING SPINE INDICATE ABNORMALITY.

• ROTATE THE TRANSDUCER 90 DEGREES TO TRAVERSE THE SPINE. THE NORMAL SPINE APPEARS AS A CLOSED CIRCLE. BEGINNING AT THE SKULL MOVE INFERIORLY ALONG THE SPINE THROUGH THE THORACIC CAVITY. NOTE THE FETAL HEART AND LUNGS.

• CONTINUE TO MOVE INFERIORLY ALONG THE SPINE INTO AND THROUGH THE ABDOMINOPELVIC CAVITY TO THE SACRUM.

NOTE THE FETAL LIVER, IVC, AORTA, KIDNEYS, AND ADRENAL GLANDS. ALSO EVALUATE THE UMBILICAL CORD AND INSERTION SITE. THE STOMACH, GALLBLADDER, AND URINARY BLADDER CAN BE EXAMINED IF FLUID-FILLED. NOTE THE BOWEL. AT THE LEVEL OF THE SACRUM LOOK FOR THE GENITALIA.

• LOCATE THE LONG AXIS OF THE FETAL SPINE AGAIN AND SCAN SUPERIORLY THROUGH TO THE BASE OF THE SKULL. SCAN THROUGH THE FETAL CRANIUM UNTIL YOU ARE BEYOND IT.

NOTE THE CONTOUR OF THE CRANIUM, INTRACRANIAL ANATOMY, AND ANY FACIAL FEATURES.

• RETURN TO THE BASE OF THE SKULL AND ROTATE THE TRANSDUCER 90 DEGREES. AGAIN SCAN THROUGH THE FETAL CRANIUM UNTIL YOU ARE BEYOND IT.

NOTE THE CONTOUR OF THE CRANIUM AND INTRACRANIAL ANATOMY.

REQUIRED PICTURES

Early First Trimester: Gestational Sac/Embryo

LONGITUDINAL IMAGES

Sagittal Plane/Anterior Approach

NOTE: Images of the gestational sac with measurements are taken whether an embryo is identified or not. Depending on how early the gestation is, it may be helpful to magnify the field of view for the gestational sac images.

1. LONG AXIS IMAGE OF THE UTERUS SHOWING THE LOCATION OF THE GESTATIONAL SAC.

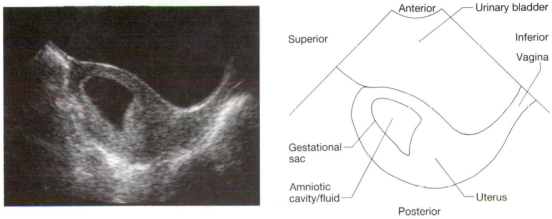

(Image courtesy of the Department of Radiology, Section of Ultrasound, Duke University Medical Center.)

LABELED: UTERUS SAG LONG AXIS

2. LONGITUDINAL IMAGE OF THE GESTATIONAL SAC WITH *SUPERIOR TO INFERIOR MEASUREMENT (CALIPERS INSIDE WALL TO INSIDE WALL).*

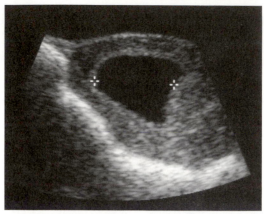

(Image courtesy of the Department of Radiology, Section of Ultrasound, Duke University Medical Center.)

LABELED: GS SAG

3. SAME IMAGE AS NUMBER 2 WITHOUT CALIPERS.

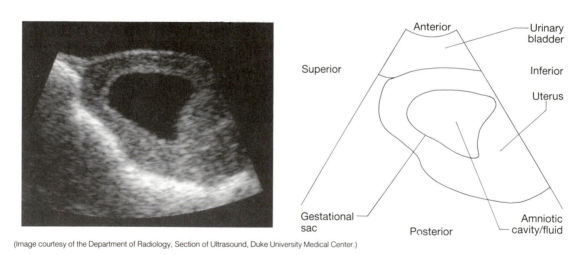

(Image courtesy of the Department of Radiology, Section of Ultrasound, Duke University Medical Center.)

LABELED: GS SAG

TRANSVERSE IMAGES

Transverse Plane/Anterior Approach

4. TRANSVERSE IMAGE OF THE GESTATIONAL SAC WITH *ANTERIOR TO POSTERIOR AND RIGHT TO LEFT MEASUREMENT (CALIPERS INSIDE WALL TO INSIDE WALL).*

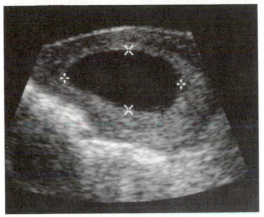

(Image courtesy of the Department of Radiology, Section of Ultrasound, Duke University Medical Center.)

LABELED: GS TRV

5. SAME IMAGE AS NUMBER 4 WITHOUT CALIPERS.

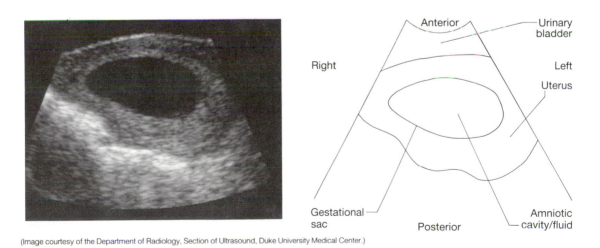

(Image courtesy of the Department of Radiology, Section of Ultrasound, Duke University Medical Center.)

LABELED: GS TRV

NOTE: If an embryo is present but not clearly represented on the gestational sac measurement images, an additional image of the embryo should be taken here and labeled accordingly.

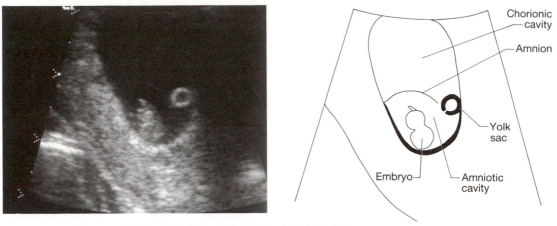

(Image courtesy of the Department of Radiology, Section of Ultrasound, Duke University Medical Center.)

First Trimester: Gestational Sac and Fetus

LONGITUDINAL IMAGES

Sagittal Plane/Anterior Approach

1. LONG AXIS IMAGE OF THE UTERUS SHOWING THE LOCATION OF THE GESTATIONAL SAC.

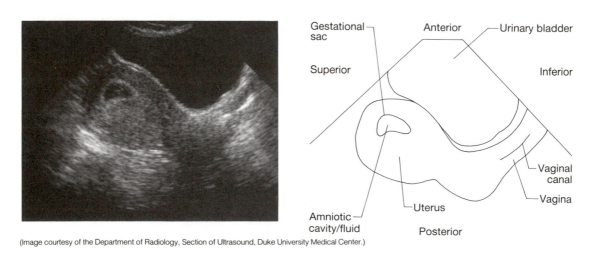

(Image courtesy of the Department of Radiology, Section of Ultrasound, Duke University Medical Center.)

LABELED: UTERUS SAG LONG AXIS

2. LONGITUDINAL IMAGE OF THE GESTATIONAL SAC TO INCLUDE THE FETUS AND PLACENTA LOCATION (IF DISTINGUISHABLE).

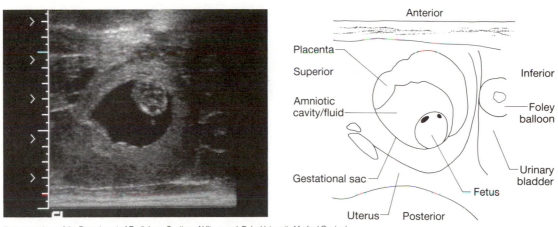

(Image courtesy of the Department of Radiology, Section of Ultrasound, Duke University Medical Center.)

LABELED: GS SAG

TRANSVERSE IMAGE

Transverse Plane/Anterior Approach

3. TRANSVERSE IMAGE OF THE GESTATIONAL SAC TO INCLUDE THE FETUS AND PLACENTA LOCATION (IF DISTINGUISHABLE).

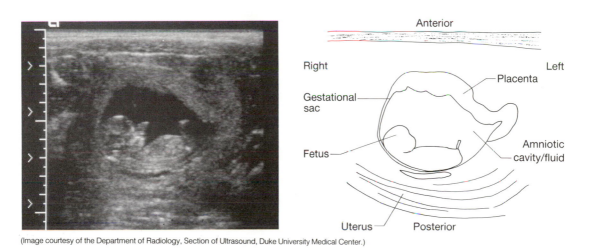

(Image courtesy of the Department of Radiology, Section of Ultrasound, Duke University Medical Center.)

LABELED: GS TRV

4. LONGITUDINAL IMAGE OF THE FETUS WITH *MEASUREMENT FROM FETAL CROWN TO RUMP.*

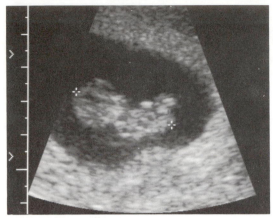

(Image courtesy of the Department of Radiology, Section of Ultrasound, Duke University Medical Center.)

LABELED: CR

NOTE: Because of the variability of the position of the fetus, scanning plane is not included as part of the film labeling on fetal measurement images.

5. SAME IMAGE AS NUMBER 4 WITHOUT CALIPERS.

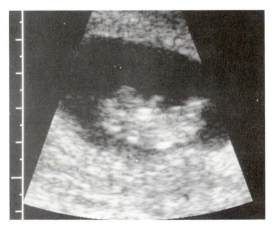 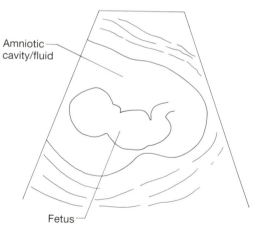

Amniotic cavity/fluid

Fetus

(Image courtesy of the Department of Radiology, Section of Ultrasound, Duke University Medical Center.)

LABELED: CR

NOTE: Depending on how early the gestation is, it may be helpful to magnify the field of view for the gestational sac and fetus.

NOTE: During the later part of the first trimester, measurements should include biparietal diameter, abdominal circumference, and other fetal measurements. See specifics for second and third trimester measurement images.

Second and Third Trimester

NOTE: Because of the variability of fetal position and movement, the following images may be taken in any sequence.

   1. WHEN THE TRIMESTER ALLOWS: LONG AXIS IMAGE OF THE UTERUS AND CONTENTS.

LABELED: UTERUS SAG LONG AXIS

NOTE: In this case the trimester was too advanced to image the entire uterus on a single view.

   2. LONGITUDINAL IMAGE OF PLACENTA LOCATION.

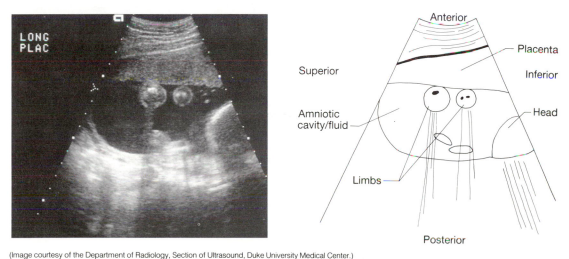

(Image courtesy of the Department of Radiology, Section of Ultrasound, Duke University Medical Center.)

LABELED: PLACENTA SAG

3. TRANSVERSE IMAGE OF PLACENTA LOCATION.

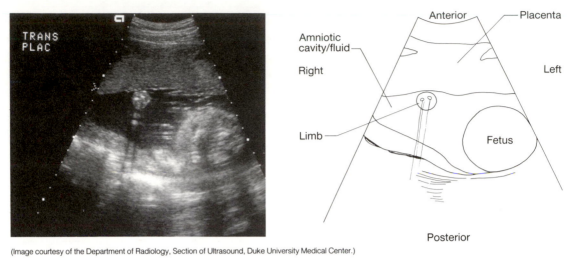

(Image courtesy of the Department of Radiology, Section of Ultrasound, Duke University Medical Center.)

LABELED: PLACENTA TRV

4. LONGITUDINAL IMAGE OF THE CERVIX TO INCLUDE THE INTERNAL OS.

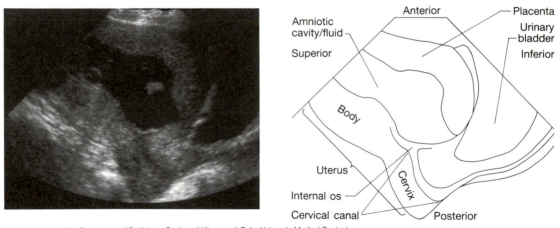

(Image courtesy of the Department of Radiology, Section of Ultrasound, Duke University Medical Center.)

LABELED: CERVX SAG

5. DEPENDING ON THE STAGE OF GESTATION, AN OVERALL LONGITUDI-NAL IMAGE OF AMNIOTIC FLUID OR THE LARGEST POCKET WITH *SUPERIOR TO INFERIOR MEASUREMENT.*

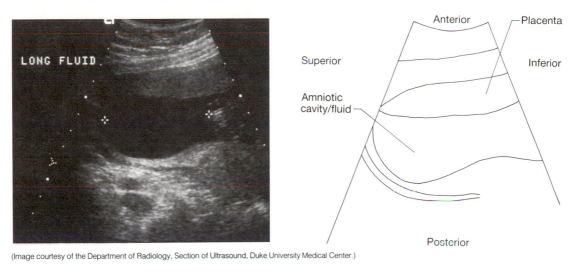

(Image courtesy of the Department of Radiology, Section of Ultrasound, Duke University Medical Center.)

LABELED: FLUID SAG

6. DEPENDING ON THE STAGE OF GESTATION, AN OVERALL TRANSVERSE IMAGE OF AMNIOTIC FLUID OR THE LARGEST POCKET WITH *ANTERIOR TO POSTERIOR AND RIGHT TO LEFT MEASUREMENTS.*

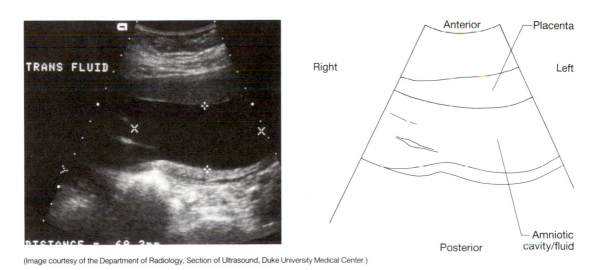

(Image courtesy of the Department of Radiology, Section of Ultrasound, Duke University Medical Center.)

LABELED: FLUID TRV

NOTE: Because of the variability of the position of the fetus, the scanning plane is not included as part of the film labeling.

7. LONGITUDINAL IMAGE OF THE CERVICAL SPINE.

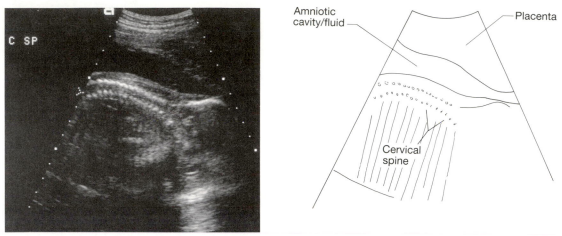

(Image courtesy of the Department of Radiology, Section of Ultrasound, Duke University Medical Center.)

LABELED: C-SPINE

8. LONGITUDINAL IMAGE OF THE THORACIC SPINE.

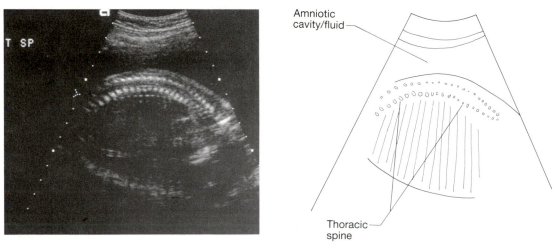

(Image courtesy of the Department of Radiology, Section of Ultrasound, Duke University Medical Center.)

LABELED: T-SPINE

9. LONGITUDINAL IMAGE OF THE LUMBAR SPINE.

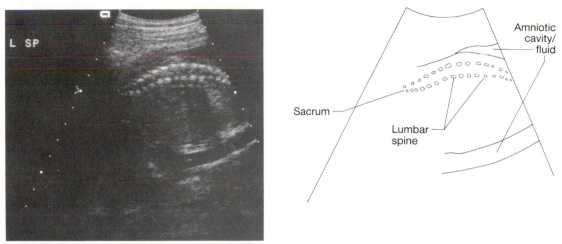

(Image courtesy of the Department of Radiology, Section of Ultrasound, Duke University Medical Center.)

LABELED: L-SPINE

NOTE: In some cases the entire spine can be imaged. If so, take the image and label: **SPINE.**

10. TRANSVERSE IMAGE OF THE CERVICAL SPINE.

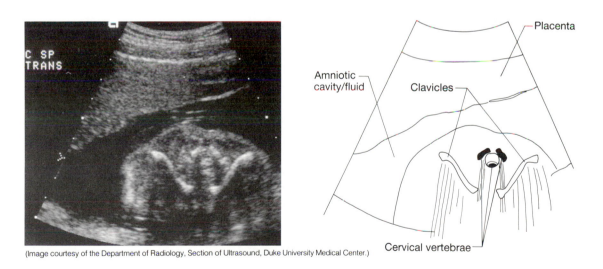

(Image courtesy of the Department of Radiology, Section of Ultrasound, Duke University Medical Center.)

LABELED: C-SPINE

11. TRANSVERSE IMAGE OF THE THORACIC SPINE.

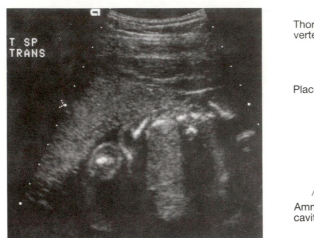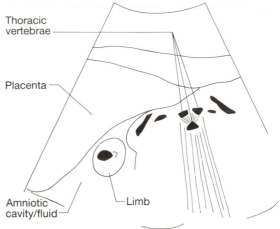

(Image courtesy of the Department of Radiology, Section of Ultrasound, Duke University Medical Center.)

LABELED: T-SPINE

12. TRANSVERSE IMAGE OF THE LUMBAR SPINE.

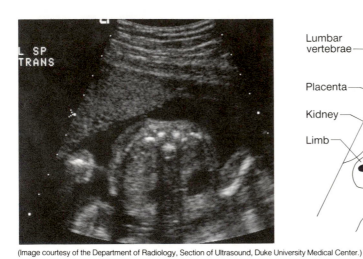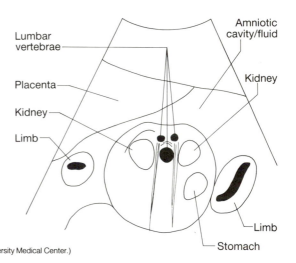

(Image courtesy of the Department of Radiology, Section of Ultrasound, Duke University Medical Center.)

LABELED: L-SPINE

13. **FOUR-CHAMBER VIEW OF THE FETAL HEART TO INCLUDE ITS LOCATION WITHIN THE THORAX.**

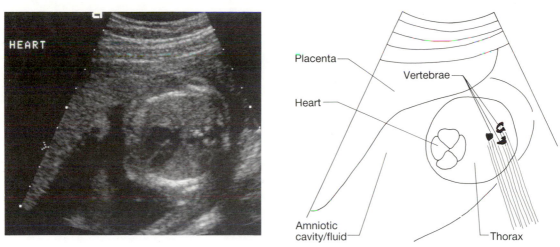

(Image courtesy of the Department of Radiology, Section of Ultrasound, Duke University Medical Center.)

LABELED: HEART

14. **TRANSVERSE IMAGE TO INCLUDE BOTH FETAL KIDNEYS IF POSSIBLE.**

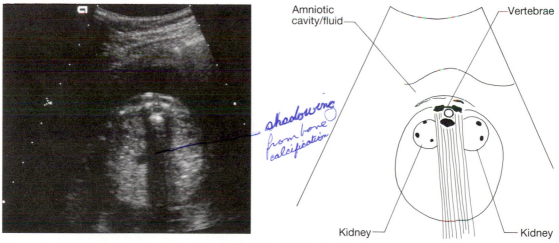

(Image courtesy of the Department of Radiology, Section of Ultrasound, Duke University Medical Center.)

LABELED: KIDNEYS

NOTE: When the kidneys cannot be imaged together because of fetal position or movement, take separate transverse images of each kidney and label accordingly.

15. LONGITUDINAL IMAGE OF THE RIGHT KIDNEY.

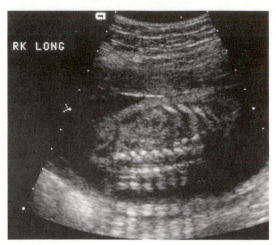

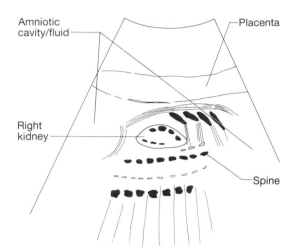

(Image courtesy of the Department of Radiology, Section of Ultrasound, Duke University Medical Center.)

LABELED: RT KID

16. LONGITUDINAL IMAGE OF THE LEFT KIDNEY.

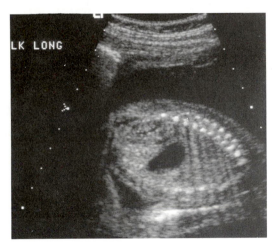

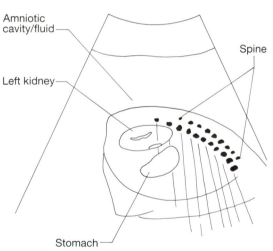

(Image courtesy of the Department of Radiology, Section of Ultrasound, Duke University Medical Center.)

LABELED: LT KID

17. IMAGE OF THE URINARY BLADDER.

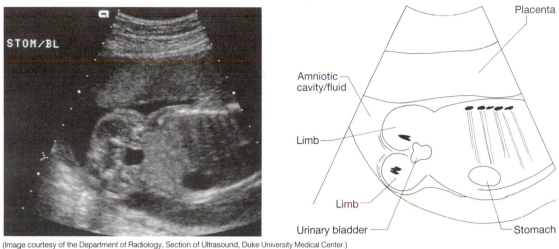

(Image courtesy of the Department of Radiology, Section of Ultrasound, Duke University Medical Center.)

LABELED: UR BLADDER

18. IMAGE OF THE UMBILICAL CORD INSERTION SITE ON THE ANTERIOR ABDOMINAL WALL.

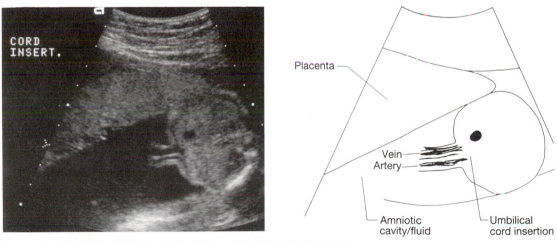

(Image courtesy of the Department of Radiology, Section of Ultrasound, Duke University Medical Center.)

LABELED: CORD

NOTE: If the insertion site image does not distinguish the three vessels of the cord, take an additional image and label accordingly.

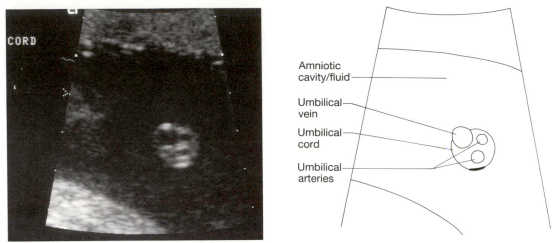

(Image courtesy of the Department of Radiology, Section of Ultrasound, Duke University Medical Center.)

LABELED: CORD

19. IMAGE OF THE STOMACH IF VISUALIZED.

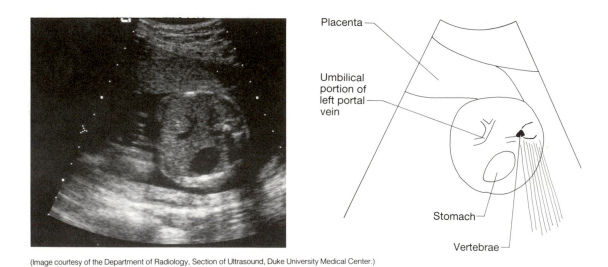

(Image courtesy of the Department of Radiology, Section of Ultrasound, Duke University Medical Center.)

LABELED: STOMACH

NOTE: The image of the stomach is not necessary if the stomach is visualized on any other image.

20. IMAGE OF FETAL GENITALIA IF VISUALIZED.

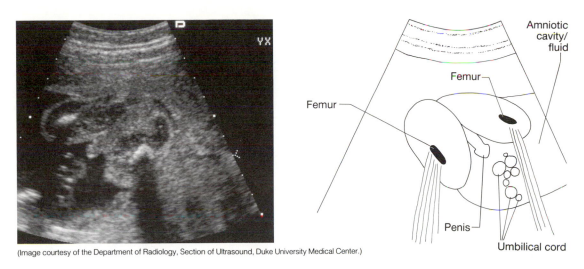

(Image courtesy of the Department of Radiology, Section of Ultrasound, Duke University Medical Center.)

LABELED: GENITALIA

21. LONGITUDINAL IMAGE OF THE FETUS TO INCLUDE THE DIAPHRAGM.

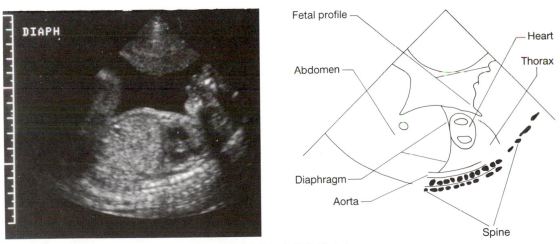

(Image courtesy of the Department of Radiology, Section of Ultrasound, Duke University Medical Center.)

LABELED: DIAPHRAGM

NOTE: Because of the obvious nature of the fetal measurements, specifics are not included as part of the film labeling.

22. BIPARIETAL DIAMETER (BPD) IMAGE AT THE LEVEL OF THE THALAMUS AND CAVUM SEPTI PELLUCIDI. *MEASUREMENT IS FROM THE INSIDE OF ONE LATERAL CRANIUM WALL TO THE OUTSIDE OF THE OTHER LATERAL CRANIUM WALL.*

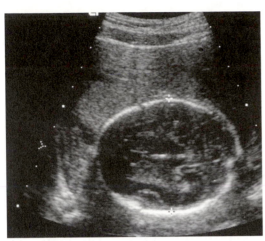 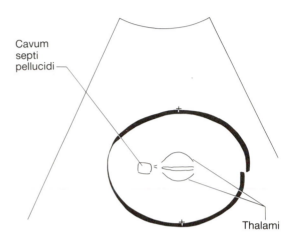

(Image courtesy of the Department of Radiology, Section of Ultrasound, Duke University Medical Center.)

23. HEAD CIRCUMFERENCE IMAGE AT THE SAME LEVEL AS THE BIPARIETAL DIAMETER OR USE THE BPD IMAGE. *MEASUREMENT IS AROUND THE OUTLINE OF THE CRANIUM.* UP-TO-DATE ULTRASOUND EQUIPMENT PROVIDES TRACKING BALLS TO TRACE THE CRANIUM OR CALIPERS THAT OPEN TO OUTLINE THE CRANIUM.

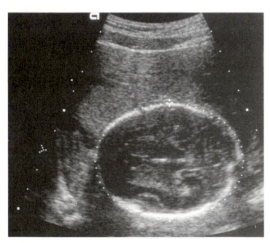 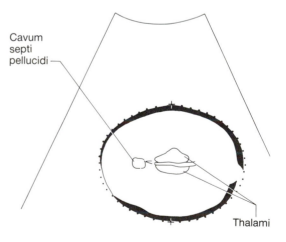

(Image courtesy of the Department of Radiology, Section of Ultrasound, Duke University Medical Center.)

24. ABDOMINAL CIRCUMFERENCE IMAGE AT THE LEVEL OF THE JUNCTION OF THE UMBILICAL VEIN AND PORTAL VEIN SINUS. *MEASUREMENT IS AROUND THE OUTLINE OF THE ABDOMEN.* THE ABDOMEN SHOULD APPEAR ROUND.

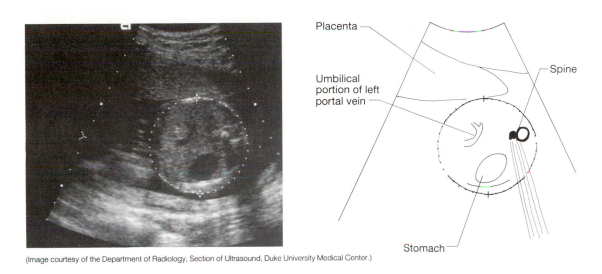

(Image courtesy of the Department of Radiology, Section of Ultrasound, Duke University Medical Center.)

25. LONG AXIS IMAGE OF THE FETAL FEMUR. *MEASUREMENT IS FROM ONE END OF THE FEMUR TO THE OTHER.*

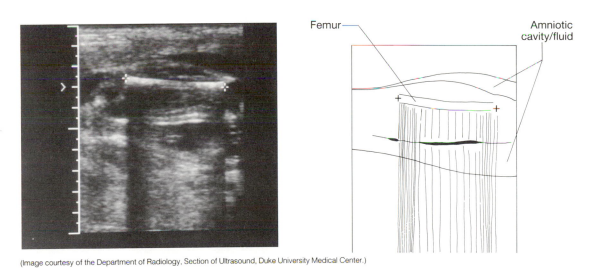

(Image courtesy of the Department of Radiology, Section of Ultrasound, Duke University Medical Center.)

NOTE: If the pregnancy is multiple, additional images are required for all trimesters that include the number of gestational sacs, number of placentae, and an image of the interposing membrane if it is present.

ENDOVAGINAL SONOGRAPHY

- Endovaginal sonography is used during the first timester when the transabdominal scan does not provide definitive information.

- Endovaginal sonography is used during the second and third trimesters to evaluate placental location in relation to the internal os of the cervix.

- See Chapter 13 for scanning method specifics.

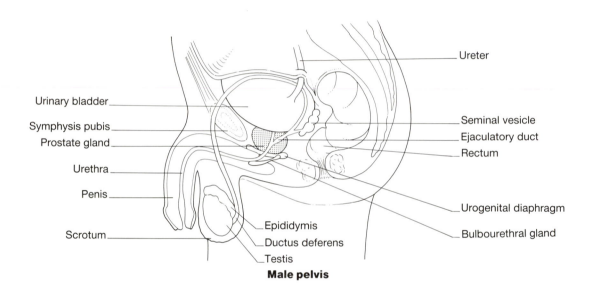

Ureter

Urinary bladder

Symphysis pubis

Prostate gland

Seminal vesicle

Ejaculatory duct

Rectum

Urethra

Penis

Urogenital diaphragm

Bulbourethral gland

Scrotum

Epididymis

Ductus deferens

Testis

Male pelvis

CHAPTER FIFTEEN

MALE PELVIS SCANNING PROTOCOL

ENDORECTAL SONOGRAPHY

- Transabdominal male pelvis examinations are rarely performed anymore. The prostate gland is the primary interest of the male pelvis and is better evaluated by endorectal sonography.

- Male pelvis transabdominal studies are systematically evaluated and documented in the same manner as the female pelvis transabdominal studies. Longitudinal surveys extend from one side of the pelvic cavity to the other. Transverse surveys extend from the symphysis pubis to the umbilicus. The prostate gland is examined from an inferior transducer angle at the level of the symphysis pubis. Patient prep, patient position, and transducer are the same as those for the female pelvis. See Chapter 13 for specifics.

LOCATION

- The urinary bladder is posterior to the symphysis pubis.

- The prostate gland is retroperitoneal. It lies anterior to the rectum and inferior to the urinary bladder.

ANATOMY

- The prostate gland is about the size of a chestnut and conical in shape. It is approximately 3.5 cm long, 4.0 cm wide, and 2.5 cm anterior to posterior. The base, its broadest aspect, is superior to its apex.

- The prostate consists of fibromuscular and glandular tissue that surrounds the neck of the bladder and urethra.

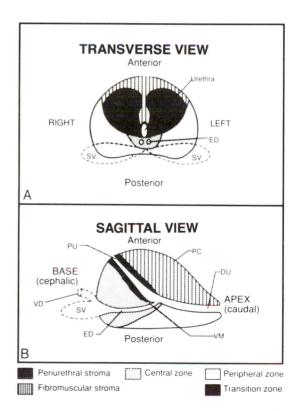

Sketches of transverse (*A*) and sagittal (*B*) views of normal prostate anatomy. Seminal vesicle (SV), verumontanum (VM), vas deferens (VD), ejaculatory duct (ED), prostatic capsule (PC), proximal urethra (PU), distal urethra (DU). (Modification of illustrations by McNeal. From Journal of Diagnostic Medical Sonography, 5:2, January/February, 1989.)

- The seminal vesicles are two sac-like structures that lie superior to the prostate and posterior to the bladder. Size is variable.

- The seminal vesicles join the vas deferens to form the ejaculatory ducts.

- The ejaculatory ducts enter the base of the prostate and pass through to the prostatic urethra at the verumontanum.

- The urethra runs from the neck of the bladder through the prostate to the base of the penis. The proximal portion of the prostatic urethra extends from the bladder neck to the verumontanum and the distal portion extends from the verumontanum to the apex of the prostate.

- The verumontanum is the area where the ejaculatory ducts join the urethra.

- The glandular portion of the prostate is divided into zones:

  - Peripheral zone: located posterior and lateral to the distal prostatic urethra. Normally, it is the largest zone.

  - Central zone: extends from the base of the prostate to the verumontanum and surrounds the ejaculatory ducts.

  - Transition zone: located on both sides of the proximal urethra. Normally, it is the smallest zone.

PHYSIOLOGY

- The function of the male reproductive organs is reproduction.

SONOGRAPHIC APPEARANCE

- The majority of the parenchyma of the prostate gland appears as midgray medium level echoes with even texture. The periurethral glandular stroma that surrounds the urethra is slightly hypoechoic compared with surrounding tissue. The contour of the gland should appear smooth and the margins well defined. Calcifications may be seen throughout the gland in older patients. The normal prostate should appear symmetrical.

- The seminal vesicles appear as symmetrical midgray or medium to low level echo textures, superior to the prostate. They are easier to visualize when the urinary bladder is partially filled. They are seen in long axis on transverse scans.

- The prostatic urethra walls appear echogenic at the midline of the gland.

- The vas deferens and ejaculatory ducts may be difficult to distinguish from surrounding structures. However, when seen, the vas deferens are medial to, and have an echo texture similar to, the seminal vesicles. The ejaculatory ducts will appear as echogenic double lines.

- Normally, the central and transition zones are not sonographically distinctive. The peripheral zone appears homogeneous and slightly hyperechoic to adjacent parenchyma.

PATIENT PREP

- Self-administered enema prior to the exam. If for some reason the patient cannot have the enema, still attempt the exam.

- Explain the examination to the patient. Verbal or written consent is required and the exam should be witnessed by another health care professional. Note that the initials of the witness should be included as part of the film labeling.

- The transducer may be inserted by the sonographer or physician.

Patient Position

- **Left lateral decubitus with knees bent toward the chest.**

- Lithotomy position.

Transducer

- **5 to 10 MHz.**

- Preparing the transducer includes providing a water path. Preparation options include:

  - Some transducer manufacturers provide a finger-like sheath that slides onto the transducer head. The sheath is secured by a small rubber band, and 20 or 30 ml of nonionized water is injected into the sheath through a pathway inside the transducer handle. Tip the transducer down and tap the water-filled sheath so any air bubbles rise to the top and can be aspirated. Fill a condom half full with sonographic gel, then put the sheathed transducer in it. Apply additional lubrication to the outside of the condom before insertion. A small rubber hose can be attached to the transducer pathway to introduce or aspirate water from the sheath to adjust for any air bubbles that might occur and cause artifacts.

  - Apply gel to the end of the transducer, then cover it with a condom. Secure the condom with a rubber band and make sure there are no air bubbles at the tip. Apply additional lubrication to the outside of the condom before insertion. Use an inner balloon filled with 30 to 50 ml of nonionized water as a water path.

  - Cover a transducer with a condom and secure it with a rubber band. Lubricate the outside of the condom, then insert the transducer into the rectum. Fill the condom with 30 to 50 ml of nonionized water for a water path.

ORIENTATION

- Sagittal and transverse views of the prostate are obtained.

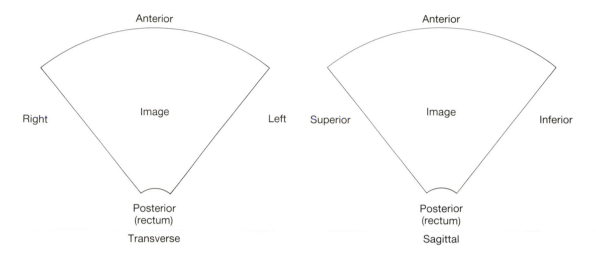

PROSTATE SURVEY

NOTE: While surveying the prostate evaluate the periprostatic fat and vessels for asymmetry and disruption in echogenicity. Also evaluate the perirectal space for pathology.

TRANSVERSE SURVEY

Transverse Plane/Rectal Approach

NOTE: To survey the prostate transversely, the transducer is inserted into the rectum and then withdrawn sequentially to examine the prostate superiorly (base) to inferiorly (apex).

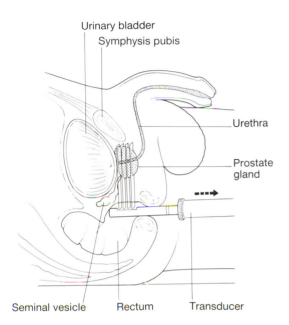

Urinary bladder
Symphysis pubis
Urethra
Prostate gland
Seminal vesicle   Rectum   Transducer

● WITH THE TRANSDUCER INSERTED THE SURVEY BEGINS AT THE LEVEL OF THE SEMINAL VESICLES.
● AFTER THE SEMINAL VESICLES AND VAS DEFERENS HAVE BEEN EVALUATED, SLOWLY WITHDRAW THE TRANSDUCER TO SCAN THROUGH THE PROSTATE FROM ITS SUPERIOR TO INFERIOR MARGINS. THE LATERAL MARGINS SHOULD BE WELL DEFINED.
    NOTE THE SIZE, SHAPE, AND SYMMETRY OF THE PROSTATE.

LONGITUDINAL SURVEY

Sagittal Plane/Rectal Approach

NOTE: To survey the prostate longitudinally the transducer is rotated clockwise, and counterclockwise to examine the prostate from one lateral edge to the other.

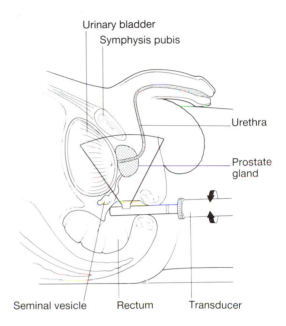

Urinary bladder
Symphysis pubis
Urethra
Prostate gland
Seminal vesicle   Rectum   Transducer

● BEGIN AT THE MIDLINE OF THE PROSTATE. THE SUPERIOR AND INFERIOR MARGINS SHOULD BE WELL DEFINED AND THE PROSTATIC URETHRA VISUALIZED.
● TO EXAMINE THE LATERAL ASPECTS OF THE PROSTATE, SEMINAL VESICLES, AND VAS DEFERENS, ROTATE THE TRANSDUCER CLOCKWISE AND COUNTERCLOCKWISE.

REQUIRED PICTURES*

TRANSVERSE IMAGES

Transverse Plane/Rectal Approach

1. TRANSVERSE IMAGE OF THE SEMINAL VESICLES.

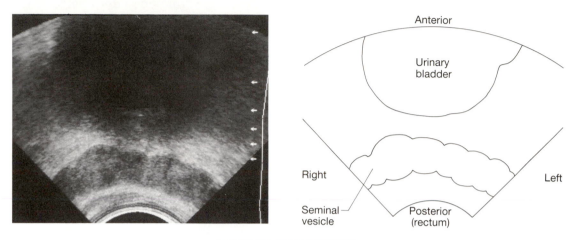

LABELED: ER TRV SEM V
("ER" INDICATES ENDORECTAL)

NOTE: Because of the limited field of view both seminal vesicles may not be entirely visible on a single view. If so, take these additional images:

2. TRANSVERSE IMAGE OF THE RIGHT SEMINAL VESICLE TO INCLUDE ITS RIGHT LATERAL MARGIN.

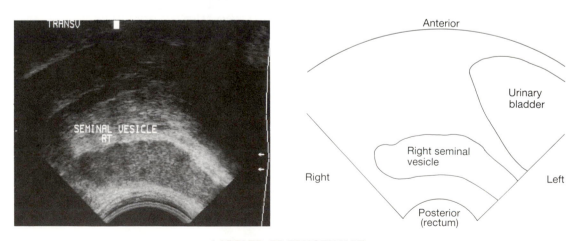

LABELED: ER TRV SEM V RT

---

*Images in this section are by courtesy of the Ultrasound Department of the Methodist Hospital, Houston, Texas.

3. TRANSVERSE IMAGE OF THE LEFT SEMINAL VESICLE TO INCLUDE ITS LEFT LATERAL MARGIN.

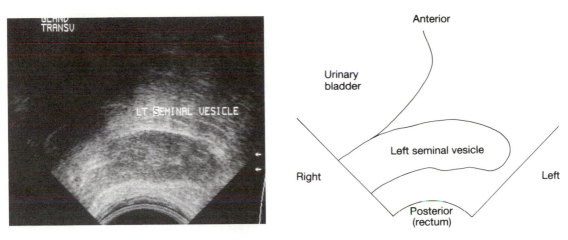

LABELED: ER TRV SEM V LT

4. TRANSVERSE IMAGE OF THE BASE OF THE PROSTATE.

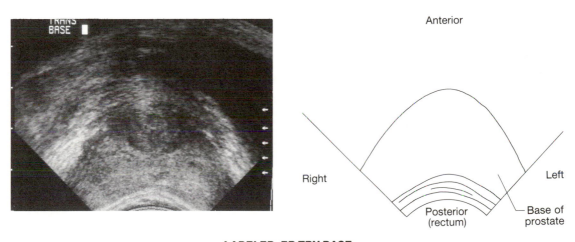

LABELED: ER TRV BASE

5. TRANSVERSE IMAGE OF THE MID PROSTATE.

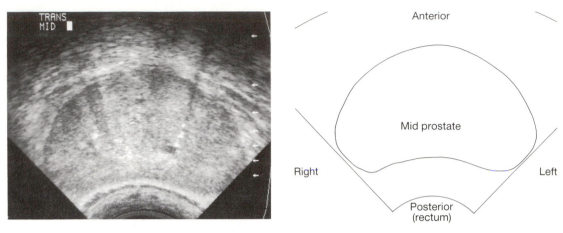

LABELED: ER TRV MID

6. TRANSVERSE IMAGE OF THE APEX OF THE PROSTATE.

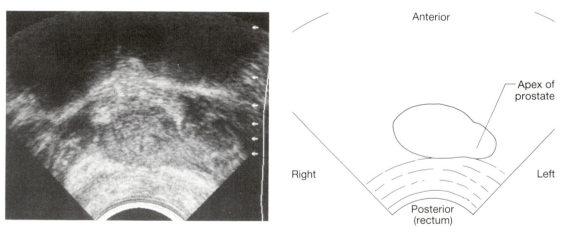

LABELED: ER TRV APEX

LONGITUDINAL IMAGES

Sagittal Plane/Rectal Approach

7. LONGITUDINAL MIDLINE IMAGE OF THE PROSTATE.

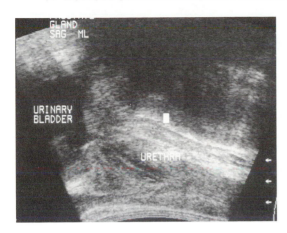 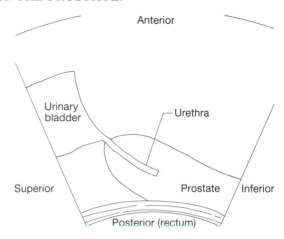

LABELED: ER SAG ML

8. LONGITUDINAL IMAGE OF THE RIGHT LATERAL PORTION OF THE PROS-
   TATE GLAND AND SEMINAL VESICLE.

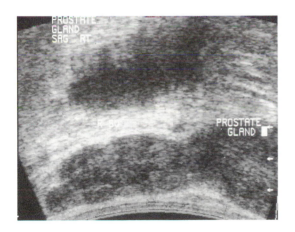 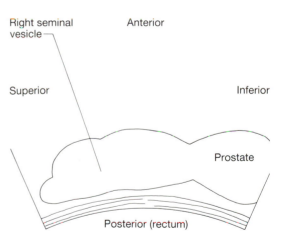

LABELED: ER SAG RT

9. LONGITUDINAL IMAGE OF THE LEFT LATERAL PORTION OF THE PROS-
   TATE GLAND AND SEMINAL VESICLE.

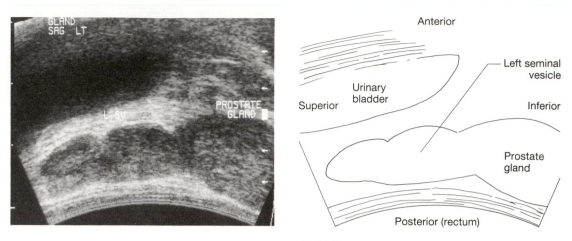

LABELED: ER SAG LT

PART IV

SMALL PARTS
SCANNING
PROTOCOLS

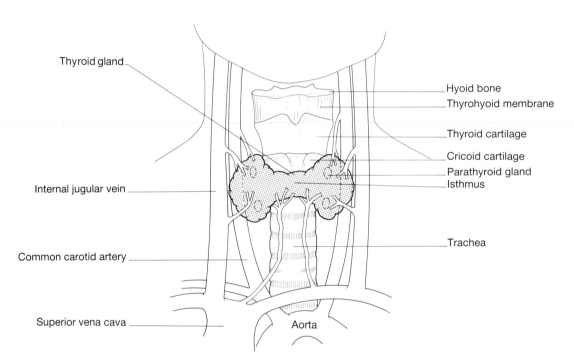

Location and anatomy of thyroid gland

Thyroid gland

Hyoid bone
Thyrohyoid membrane

Thyroid cartilage

Cricoid cartilage
Parathyroid gland
Isthmus

Internal jugular vein

Trachea

Common carotid artery

Superior vena cava

Aorta

CHAPTER SIXTEEN

THYROID GLAND SCANNING PROTOCOL

LOCATION

- Lower, anterior portion of the neck.
- The lateral borders of the lobes are the common carotid artery and internal jugular vein.
- The medial border of the lobes is the trachea.
- The isthmus lies anterior to the trachea.
- The sternocleidomastoid, sternothyroid, and sternohyoid muscles are anterior to the thyroid.
- The longus colli muscle is posterior to the thyroid.

ANATOMY

- Butterfly-shaped gland with right and left lobes.
- The right and left lobes are connected at the midline by a narrow portion of the gland called the isthmus.
- The thyroid is variable in size but weighs approximately 30 g. The thyroid is larger in women and becomes enlarged during pregnancy.
- Each lobe is approximately 5 cm long, 2 cm anterior to posterior, and 3 cm at its greatest width.
- The thyroid is a highly vascular gland with four arteries and veins.

PHYSIOLOGY

- Endocrine gland that synthesizes, stores, and secretes thyroid hormones.
- Maintains body metabolism.

SONOGRAPHIC APPEARANCE

- Lobes are midgray or medium-level echoes with even texture.

- Lobes appear more echogenic than adjacent muscles.

- Small anechoic venous structures may be seen as they course within or adjacent to the thyroid.

NORMAL VARIANTS

- Pyramidal lobe:
  Triangular-shaped, superior extension of the isthmus. Present in 15% to 30% of thyroid glands. Variable in size and extends more often to the left side. Parenchyma appears the same as the normal thyroid.

- Dilated follicles:
  Interspersed throughout the thyroid, they appear as 1- to 3-mm cystic areas.

PATIENT PREP

- None.

PATIENT POSITION

- Supine.
- Neck hyperextended by placing a sponge or pillow under the patient's neck.

TRANSDUCER

- **10 MHz.**
- 7.5 MHz recommended for a very muscular or fat neck.
- According to the transducer and machine used, a water path or standoff pad may be necessary.

BREATHING TECHNIQUE

- **Normal respiration.**

THYROID SURVEY

NOTE: The thyroid gland is small and can be seen in its entirety by some transducers, but it is still evaluated by viewing the lobes individually.

TRANSVERSE SURVEY

Transverse Plane/Anterior Approach

● BEGIN WITH THE TRANSDUCER PERPENDICULAR AT THE STERNAL NOTCH.

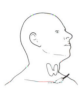

● MOVE THE TRANSDUCER SLIGHTLY SUPERIOR AND TOWARD THE PATIENT'S RIGHT, LATERAL ENOUGH TO VIEW THE RIGHT LOBE FROM ITS MEDIAL TO LATERAL MARGINS.

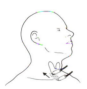

● KEEP THE TRANSDUCER PERPENDICULAR AND SCAN SUPERIORLY THROUGH AND BEYOND THE RIGHT LOBE TO THE LEVEL OF THE MANDIBLE. NOTE THE ISTHMUS MEDIALLY.

● MOVE THE TRANSDUCER INFERIORLY FROM THE MANDIBLE BACK THROUGH AND BEYOND THE INFERIOR MARGIN OF THE RIGHT LOBE TO THE LEVEL OF THE STERNAL NOTCH.

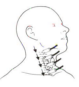

● MOVE THE TRANSDUCER SLIGHTLY SUPERIOR AND TOWARD THE PATIENT'S LEFT, LATERAL ENOUGH TO VIEW THE LEFT LOBE FROM ITS MEDIAL TO LATERAL MARGINS.

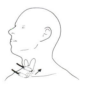

• KEEP THE TRANSDUCER PERPENDICU-LAR AND SCAN SUPERIORLY THROUGH AND BEYOND THE RIGHT LOBE TO THE LEVEL OF THE MANDIBLE. NOTE THE ISTHMUS MEDIALLY.

• MOVE THE TRANSDUCER INFERIORLY FROM THE MANDIBLE BACK THROUGH AND BEYOND THE INFERIOR MARGIN OF THE LEFT LOBE TO THE LEVEL OF THE STERNAL NOTCH.

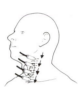

• MOVE TO THE MIDLINE OF THE STER-NAL NOTCH AND SCAN SUPERIORLY UNTIL YOU SCAN THROUGH AND BEYOND THE ISTHMUS.

LONGITUDINAL SURVEY

Sagittal Plane/Anterior Approach

• BEGIN WITH THE TRANSDUCER PER-PENDICULAR AT THE MIDLINE OF THE STERNAL NOTCH.

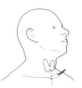

• MOVE THE TRANSDUCER SLIGHTLY SU-PERIOR AND TOWARD THE PATIENT'S RIGHT, ENOUGH TO VIEW THE RIGHT LOBE FROM ITS SUPERIOR TO INFERIOR MARGINS.

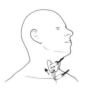

- KEEP THE TRANSDUCER PERPENDICU-LAR AND SCAN TOWARD THE PATIENT'S RIGHT, LATERALLY THROUGH AND BE-YOND THE RIGHT LOBE.

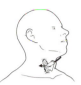

- KEEP THE TRANSDUCER PERPENDICU-LAR AND SCAN TOWARD THE PATIENT'S LEFT, LATERALLY THROUGH AND BE-YOND THE LEFT LOBE.

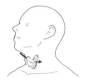

- MOVE BACK ONTO THE LOBE AND SCAN THROUGH TO THE MIDLINE AND THE ISTHMUS.

- MOVE BACK ONTO THE LOBE AND SCAN THROUGH TO THE MIDLINE AND THE ISTHMUS.

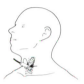

- FROM THE MIDLINE MOVE THE TRANS-DUCER SLIGHTLY TOWARD THE PA-TIENT'S LEFT, ENOUGH TO VIEW THE LEFT LOBE FROM ITS SUPERIOR TO IN-FERIOR MARGINS.

NOTE: Imaging the inferior portion of the lobes can be improved by having the patient swallow. This raises the gland superiorly.

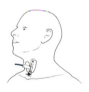

REQUIRED PICTURES

RIGHT LOBE

Transverse Images

Transverse Plane/Anterior Approach

1. TRANSVERSE IMAGE OF THE INFERIOR PORTION OF THE RIGHT LOBE.

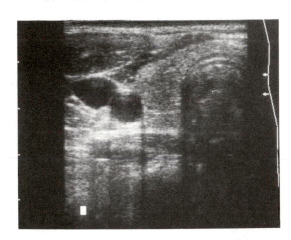 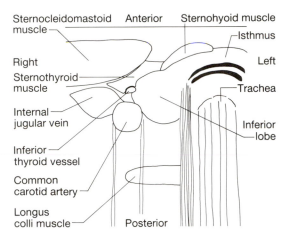

LABELED: RT LOBE TRV INF

2. TRANSVERSE IMAGE OF THE MIDPORTION OF THE RIGHT LOBE.

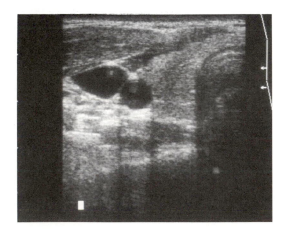 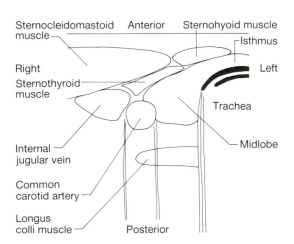

LABELED: RT LOBE TRV MID

3. TRANSVERSE IMAGE OF THE SUPERIOR PORTION OF THE RIGHT LOBE.

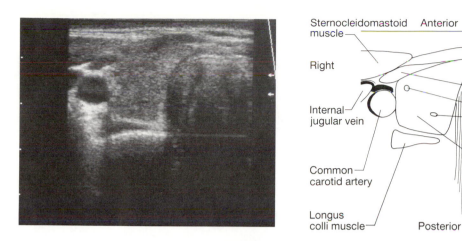

LABELED: RT LOBE TRV SUP

4. TRANSVERSE IMAGE OF THE ISTHMUS TO INCLUDE BOTH THE RIGHT AND LEFT LOBE ATTACHMENTS.

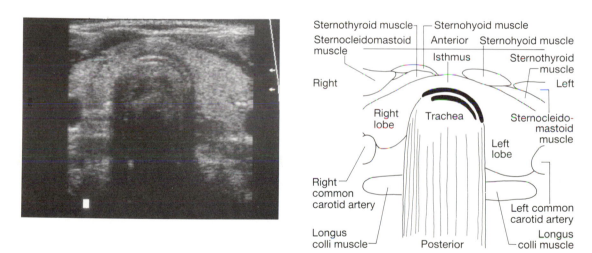

LABELED: ISTHMUS TRV

Longitudinal Images

Sagittal Plane/Anterior Approach

5. LONGITUDINAL IMAGE OF THE MEDIAL PORTION OF THE RIGHT LOBE.

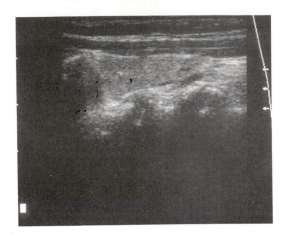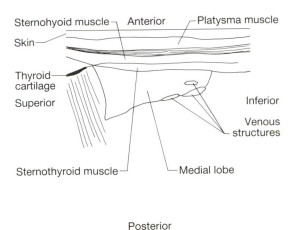

LABELED: RT LOBE SAG MED

6. LONGITUDINAL IMAGE OF THE LATERAL PORTION OF THE RIGHT LOBE.

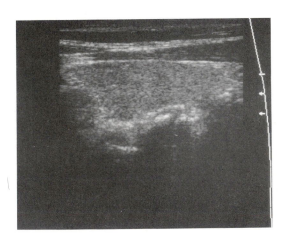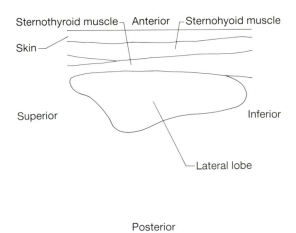

LABELED: RT LOBE SAG LAT

LEFT LOBE

Transverse Images

Transverse Plane/Anterior Approach

7. TRANSVERSE IMAGE OF THE INFERIOR PORTION OF THE LEFT LOBE.

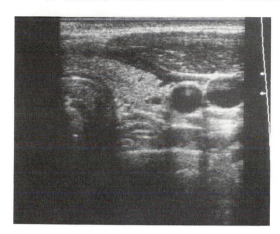 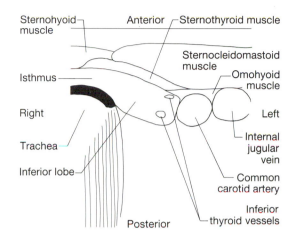

LABELED: LT LOBE TRV INF

8. TRANSVERSE IMAGE OF THE MIDPORTION OF THE LEFT LOBE.

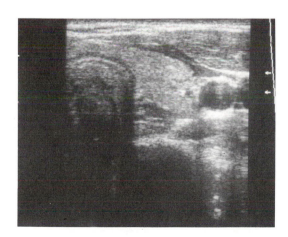 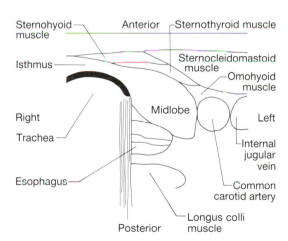

LABELED: LT LOBE TRV MID

9. TRANSVERSE IMAGE OF THE SUPERIOR PORTION OF THE LEFT LOBE.

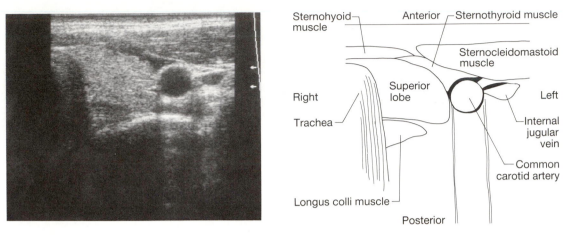

LABELED: LT LOBE TRV SUP

Longitudinal Images

Sagittal Plane/Anterior Approach

10. LONGITUDINAL IMAGE OF THE MEDIAL PORTION OF THE LEFT LOBE.

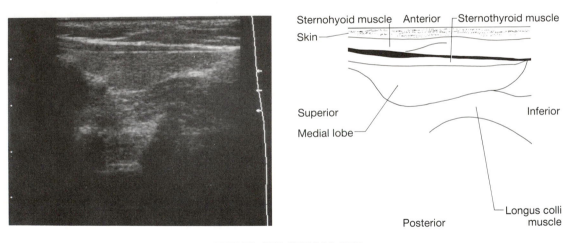

LABELED: LT LOBE SAG MED

11. LONGITUDINAL IMAGE OF THE LATERAL PORTION OF THE LEFT LOBE.

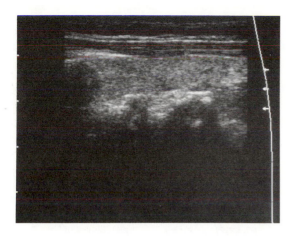

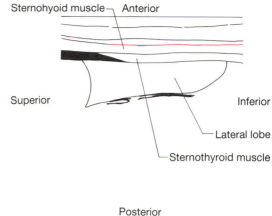

LABELED: LT LOBE SAG LAT

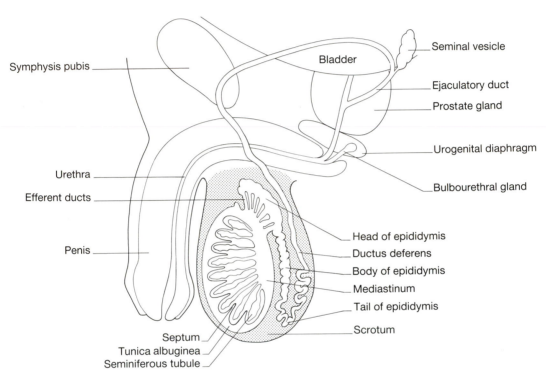

Symphysis pubis

Bladder

Seminal vesicle

Ejaculatory duct

Prostate gland

Urogenital diaphragm

Bulbourethral gland

Urethra

Efferent ducts

Penis

Head of epididymis

Ductus deferens

Body of epididymis

Mediastinum

Tail of epididymis

Scrotum

Septum

Tunica albuginea

Seminiferous tubule

Scrotum anatomy

CHAPTER SEVENTEEN
SCROTUM SCANNING PROTOCOL

ANATOMY

- A two-compartment sac divided by a septum.

- Each compartment contains a testis, epididymis, and a portion of the ductus deferens (spermatic cord).

- Testes are ovoid with the superior pole lying more anterior.

- Testes are approximately 4 to 5 cm long, and 2.5 to 3 cm wide.

- The epididymis is located at the posterosuperior and posteroinferior lateral borders of the testes.

- The epididymis is approximately 6 to 7 cm long. The diameter of the head is 7 to 8 mm, and the diameter of the tail is 1 to 2 mm.

PHYSIOLOGY

- Functions as an endocrine gland by synthesizing and secreting testosterone, the male hormone.

- Functions as an exocrine gland by producing spermatozoa.

SONOGRAPHIC APPEARANCE

- The testes appear as midgray or medium-level echoes with even texture. Testicular parenchyma is similar to that of the normal thyroid gland.

- The mediastinum testes often appear as a highly echogenic line parallel to the epididymis.

- The epididymis appears as midgray or medium-level echoes that are equal to or slightly more echogenic than the normal testes. The head is easier to visualize than the body or tail.

- It is normal to visualize 1 to 2 mm of fluid surrounding the testes.

Patient Prep

- The scrotum can be supported by a towel draped beneath it or held in the examiner's gloved hand.

- Hand-held has the advantage of allowing correlation between a palpable lesion and its sonographic findings. Also, the examiner's finger is easily identified as highly echogenic.

Patient Position

- **Supine with the legs slightly spread or in a semi–frog-legged position.**

- Upright.

Transducer

- **7.5 MHz.**

- 10 MHz.

Scrotum Survey

NOTE: Use the following survey steps for both testes.

LONGITUDINAL SURVEY

Sagittal Plane/Anterior Approach

● BEGIN WITH THE TRANSDUCER PERPENDICULAR AT MID TESTIS.

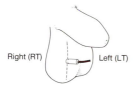

● MOVE THE TRANSDUCER MEDIALLY THROUGH AND BEYOND THE TESTIS AND SCROTAL SAC.

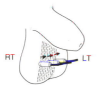

● SCAN BACK TO MID TESTIS AND MOVE THE TRANSDUCER LATERALLY THROUGH AND BEYOND THE TESTIS AND SCROTAL SAC.

NOTE: You should be able to see the entire testicle superior to inferior. If not, move the transducer superior and inferior as you scan to evaluate the enitre area (testis, epididymis, and scrotal sac).

TRANSVERSE SURVEY

Transverse Plane/Anterior Approach

● BEGIN WITH THE TRANSDUCER PERPENDICULAR AT MID TESTIS.

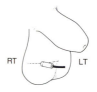

● MOVE THE TRANSDUCER SUPERIORLY THROUGH AND BEYOND THE TESTIS AND SCROTAL SAC.

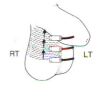

● SCAN BACK TO MID TESTIS AND MOVE THE TRANSDUCER INFERIORLY THROUGH AND BEYOND THE TESTIS AND SCROTAL SAC.

NOTE: You should be able to see the entire testicle medial to lateral. If not, move the transducer laterally and medially as you scan to evaluate the entire area (testis, epididymis, and scrotal sac).

REQUIRED PICTURES

RIGHT TESTIS

Longitudinal Images
Sagittal Plane/Anterior Approach

1. LONGITUDINAL IMAGE OF THE MIDPORTION OF THE RIGHT TESTIS.

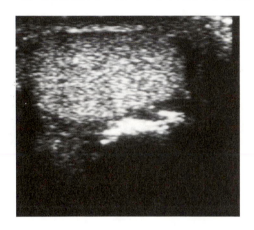
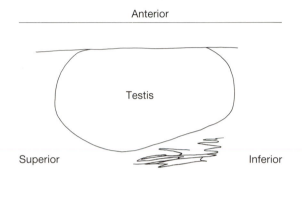

LABELED: RT TESTIS SAG MID

2. LONGITUDINAL IMAGE OF THE LATERAL PORTION OF THE RIGHT TESTIS TO INCLUDE THE EPIDIDYMIS.

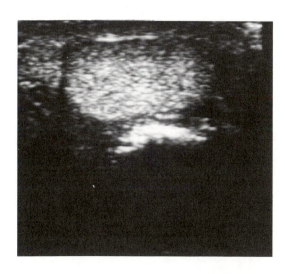
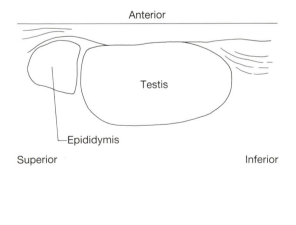

LABELED: RT TESTIS SAG LAT

3. LONGITUDINAL IMAGE OF THE MEDIAL PORTION OF THE RIGHT TESTIS.

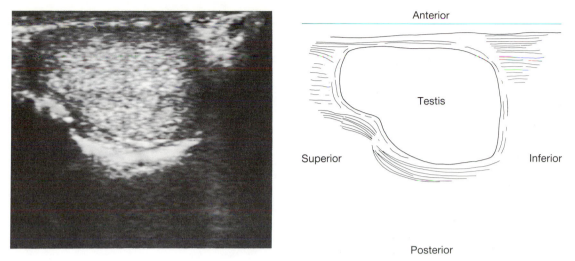

LABELED: RT TESTIS SAG MED

Transverse Images

Transverse Plane/Anterior Approach

4. TRANSVERSE IMAGE OF THE MIDPORTION OF THE RIGHT TESTIS.

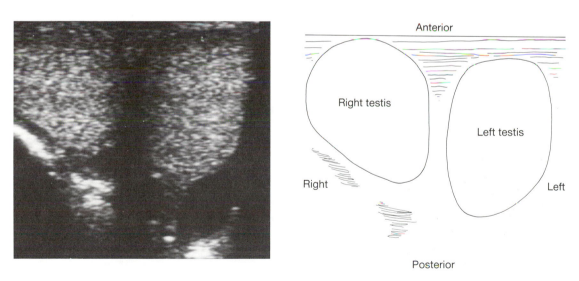

LABELED: RT TESTIS TRV MID

5. TRANSVERSE IMAGE OF THE SUPERIOR PORTION OF THE RIGHT TESTIS.

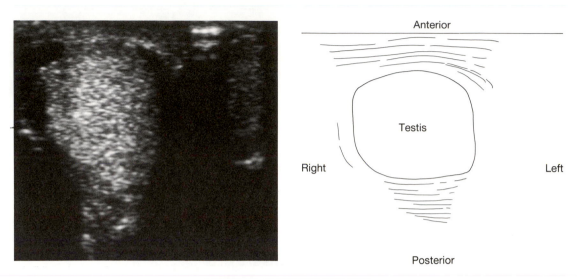

LABELED: RT TESTIS TRV SUP

6. TRANSVERSE IMAGE OF THE INFERIOR PORTION OF THE RIGHT TESTIS.

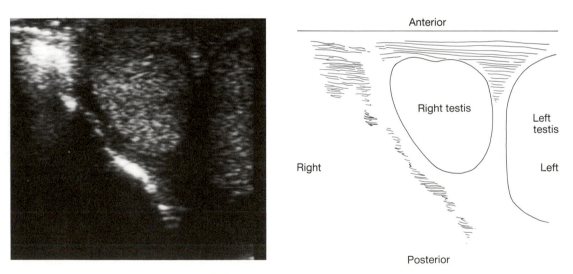

LABELED: RT TESTIS TRV INF

LEFT TESTIS

Longitudinal Images

Sagittal Plane/Anterior Approach

7. LONGITUDINAL IMAGE OF THE MIDPORTION OF THE LEFT TESTIS.

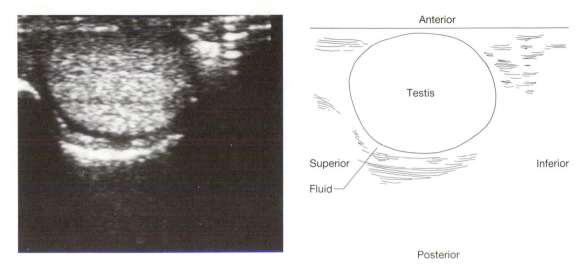

LABELED: LT TESTIS SAG MID

8. LONGITUDINAL IMAGE OF THE LATERAL PORTION OF THE LEFT TESTIS TO INCLUDE THE EPIDIDYMIS.

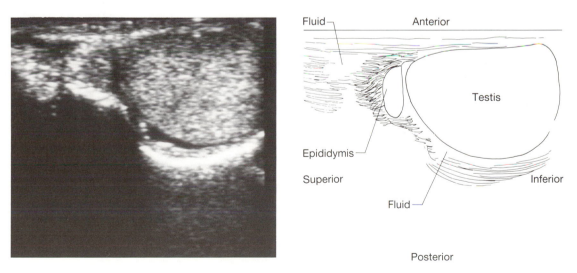

LABELED: LT TESTIS SAG LAT

9. LONGITUDINAL IMAGE OF THE MEDIAL PORTION OF THE LEFT TESTIS.

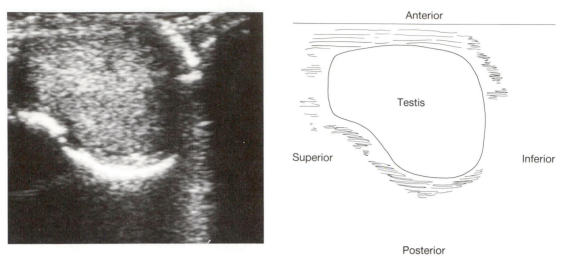

LABELED: LT TESTIS SAG MED

Transverse Images

Transverse Plane/Anterior Approach

10. TRANSVERSE IMAGE OF THE MIDPORTION OF THE LEFT TESTIS.

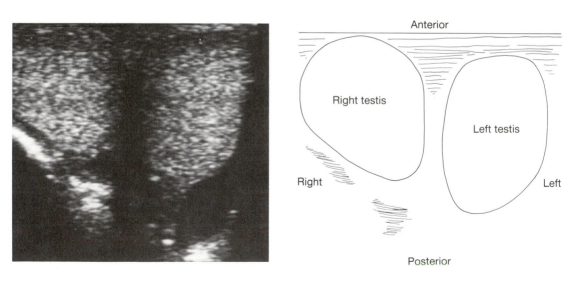

LABELED: LT TESTIS TRV MID

11. TRANSVERSE IMAGE OF THE SUPERIOR PORTION OF THE LEFT TESTIS.

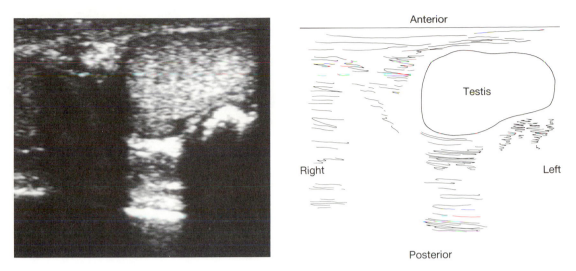

LABELED: LT TESTIS TRV SUP

12. TRANSVERSE IMAGE OF THE INFERIOR PORTION OF THE LEFT TESTIS.

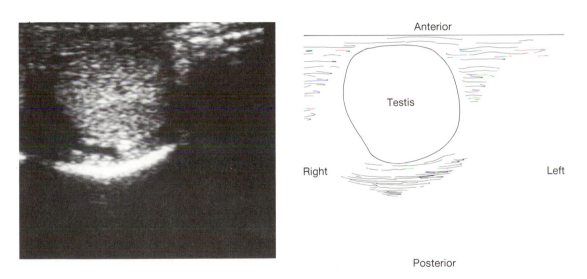

LABELED: LT TESTIS TRV INF

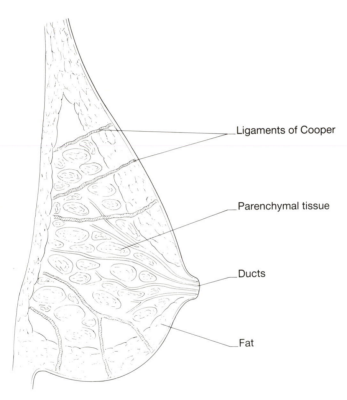

Ligaments of Cooper

Parenchymal tissue

Ducts

Fat

Breast anatomy

CHAPTER EIGHTEEN
BREAST SCANNING PROTOCOL

BETTY BATES TEMPKIN and FELICIA M. TERRY

ANATOMY

- Breast parenchymal elements are lobes, ducts, lobules, and acini.
- Most posterior aspect is connected to the pectoral musculature.
- Most anterior aspect is connected to the skin.

PHYSIOLOGY

- Mammary function is to secrete milk during lactation.

SONOGRAPHIC APPEARANCE

- The skin line, nipple, and the retromammary layer are highly echogenic.
- The areolar area is slightly less echogenic than the nipple and skin.
- Internal nipple appearance is quite variable.
- The mammary layer (active glandular tissue) is the core of the breast and has a mixed parenchymal appearance depending on the amount of fat that is present.

NOTE: Appearance with the presence of little fat is highly echogenic because of collagen and fibrotic tissue. When fat is present, the appearance is of areas of low-level echoes mixed with areas of high echogenicity.

- Cooper's ligament and other connective tissue can be seen as highly echogenic linear areas within the fat tissue.
- The sonographic appearance of the breast changes with age. Older patients' breasts tend to have more fatty tissue.

PATIENT PREP

- None.

PATIENT POSITION

- **Supine.**
- Sitting erect.

TRANSDUCER

- **5 MHz linear.**
- 7.5 MHz.
- 10 MHz.

CLINICAL REASONING

- Sonography of the breast should be performed only after mammography unless the patient is under 25 years old.
- Breast sonography is generally performed to determine the composition of a localized areas(s) that may or may not be palpable.

227

- Whole breast scanning may be indicated for diffuse diseases such as fibrocystic disease.

BREAST SURVEY

NOTE: For localized area(s) see pathology scanning protocol, Chapter 3.

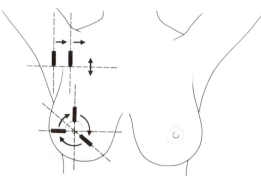

Survey reference

WHOLE BREAST SURVEY

- BEGIN SCANNING THE BREAST IN QUESTION AT THE 12 O'CLOCK POSITION.
- TRANSDUCER ORIENTATION IS SET UP SO THAT THE BREAST IS VIEWED IN SECTIONS FROM NIPPLE OUTWARD, WHERE THE ORIENTATION NOTCH IS LOCATED.
- SCAN AROUND THE BREAST IN A CLOCKWISE MANNER, COVERING ALL ANATOMY, INCLUDING THE AXILLARY REGIONS.

NOTE: If it is necessary to scan the entire breast for diffuse disease, you must scan both breasts.

REQUIRED PICTURES

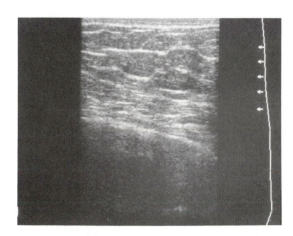

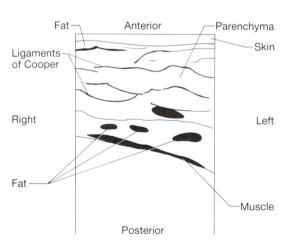

Breast image reference

1. 12 O'CLOCK IMAGE OF BREAST TISSUE WITH THE BASE OF THE TRANSDUCER TOWARD THE NIPPLE AND THE END OF THE TRANSDUCER FACING OUTWARD SO THAT THE NIPPLE AREA IS CLOSEST TO THE TOP OF THE IMAGING SCREEN.

LABELED: 12 O'CLOCK RT OR LT

2. 3 O'CLOCK IMAGE (SAME ORIENTATION AS NUMBER 1).

LABELED: 3 O'CLOCK RT OR LT

3. 6 O'CLOCK IMAGE.

LABELED: 6 O'CLOCK RT OR LT

4. 9 O'CLOCK IMAGE.

LABELED: 9 O'CLOCK RT OR LT

5. TRANSVERSE IMAGE THROUGH THE NIPPLE.

LABELED: NIP TRV RT OR LT

6. LONGITUDINAL IMAGE THROUGH THE NIPPLE.

LABELED: NIP SAG RT OR LT

7. LONGITUDINAL IMAGE OF THE AXILLARY REGION.

LABELED: AXILLARY SAG RT OR LT

8. TRANSVERSE IMAGE OF THE AXILLARY REGION.

LABELED: AXILLARY TRV RT OR LT

9 to 16. WILL BE THE SAME CORRESPONDING PICTURES OF THE OTHER BREAST.

NOTE: In some cases, whole breast scanning includes images from 12 o'clock, 1 o'clock, 2 o'clock, 3 o'clock, etc. If so, label accordingly and include nipple and axillary images.

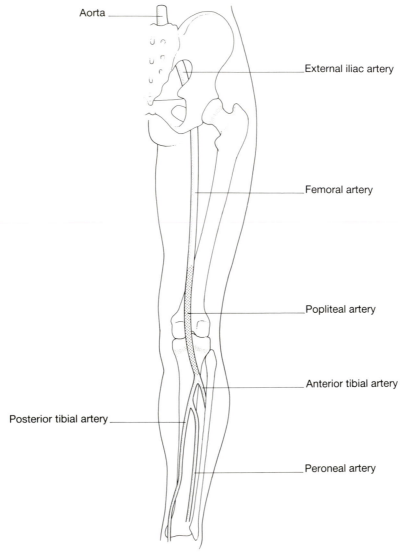

Aorta

External iliac artery

Femoral artery

Popliteal artery

Anterior tibial artery

Posterior tibial artery

Peroneal artery

(Redrawn from Kapit W, Elson LM: The Anatomy Coloring Book. New York, Harper & Row, 1977.)

Popliteal artery anatomy

CHAPTER NINETEEN

POPLITEAL ARTERY SCANNING PROTOCOL

LOCATION

- The popliteal artery courses through the popliteal fossa as it extends from the middle and lower thirds of the thigh, downward to the lower border of the popliteus where it bifurcates.

ANATOMY

- It is the continuation of the femoral artery.
- Bifurcates into the anterior and posterior tibial arteries.

PHYSIOLOGY

- Supplies oxygen and nutrient-rich blood to the lower leg.

SONOGRAPHIC APPEARANCE

- Anechoic lumen surrounded by echogenic walls.

PATIENT PREP

- None.

PATIENT POSITION

- Prone.

TRANSDUCER

- **7.5 MHz.**
- 10 MHz.

POPLITEAL ARTERY SURVEY

LONGITUDINAL SURVEY

Sagittal Plane/Posterior Approach

- BEGIN WITH THE TRANSDUCER PERPENDICULAR AT THE BEND OF THE KNEE.

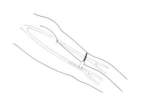

● MOVE THE TRANSDUCER SLIGHTLY MEDIAL AND INFERIOR TO LOCATE THE ARTERY. ONCE LOCATED, SLIGHTLY ROCK THE TRANSDUCER RIGHT TO LEFT, SCANNING THROUGH EACH SIDE OF THE ARTERY AS YOU ALSO MOVE SUPERIOR AND INFERIOR ALONG ITS LENGTH.

● VIEWING THE LONGITUDINAL ARTERY ROTATE THE TRANSDUCER 90 DEGREES INTO THE TRANSVERSE PLANE.

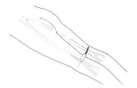

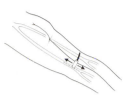

● LOOK FOR THE TRAVERSED, ROUND-APPEARING ARTERY. ONCE LOCATED, SLOWLY ROCK THE TRANSDUCER SUPERIORLY AND INFERIORLY WHILE SLIDING ALONG THE LENGTH OF THE ARTERY.

NOTE: Look for the pulsating popliteal artery lying posterior to the popliteal vein.

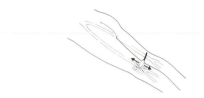

TRANSVERSE SURVEY

Transverse Plane/Posterior Approach

NOTE: Always scan the other leg's popliteal artery to compare sizes.

REQUIRED PICTURES

LONGITUDINAL IMAGES

Sagittal Plane/Posterior Approach

1. LONGITUDINAL IMAGE OF THE PROXIMAL POPLITEAL ARTERY.

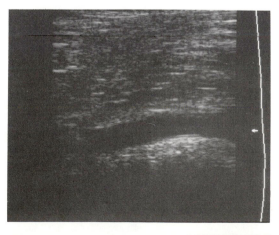

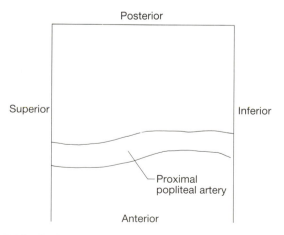

LABELED: RT OR LT POP SAG PROX

2. LONGITUDINAL IMAGE OF THE DISTAL POPLITEAL ARTERY.

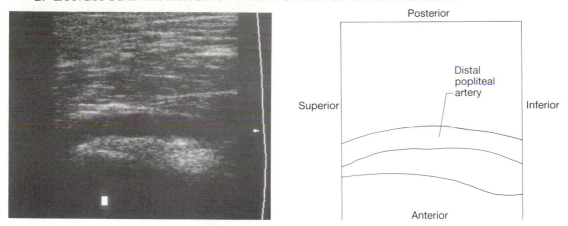

LABELED: RT OR LT POP SAG DIST

TRANSVERSE IMAGES
Transverse Plane/Posterior Approach

3. TRANSVERSE IMAGE OF THE POPLITEAL ARTERY WITH *ANTERIOR TO POSTERIOR MEASUREMENT*.

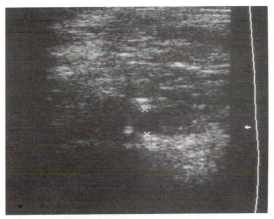

LABELED: RT OR LT POP TRV

4. SAME IMAGE AS NUMBER 3 WITHOUT CALIPERS.

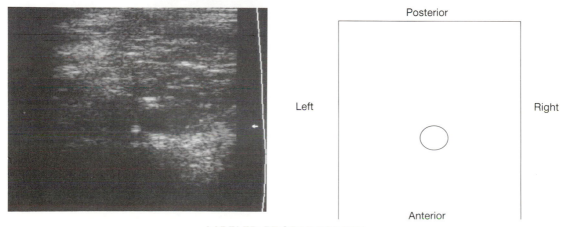

LABELED: RT OR LT POP TRV

5 to 8. WILL BE THE CORRESPONDING IMAGES OF THE OTHER LEG'S POPLI-TEAL ARTERY.

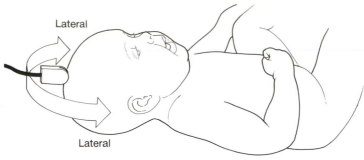

Lateral

Lateral

Sagittal

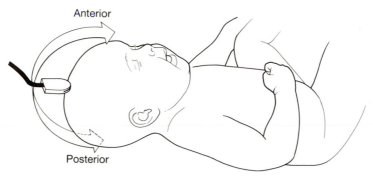

Anterior

Posterior

Coronal

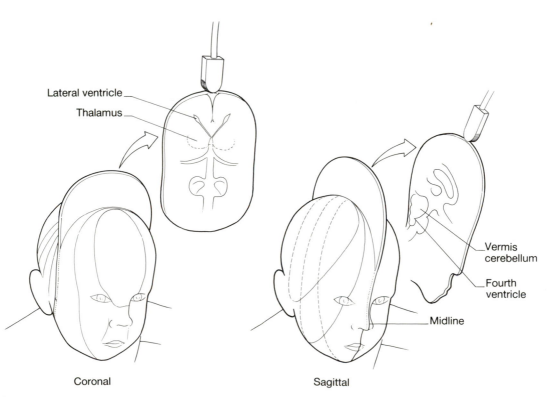

Lateral ventricle

Thalamus

Vermis cerebellum

Fourth ventricle

Midline

Coronal

Sagittal

CHAPTER TWENTY
NEONATAL BRAIN SCANNING PROTOCOL

KRISTIN DYKSTRA-DOWNEY

CRANIAL VAULT ANATOMY AND SONOGRAPHIC APPEARANCE

- Four ventricles:
  - Two lateral ventricles:
    Each ventricle is divided segmentally into a frontal horn, body, occipital horn, and temporal horn. The atrium or trigone is the junction of the body and occipital and temporal horns. The ventricle walls appear echogenic and curvilinear. These slit-like structures lie the same distance from the interhemispheric fissure. The cavities contain cerebrospinal fluid (CSF) and appear anechoic.

  - Third ventricle:
    The third ventricle is a small, tear-drop–shaped, midline cavity that lies between the thalami and is connected to the lateral ventricles via the foramen of Monro. The walls appear echogenic. The cavity contains CSF and appears anechoic.

  - Fourth ventricle:
    The fourth ventricle is a small, thin, arrowhead-shaped midline cavity that appears to project into the cerebellum. It is vaguely seen except with massive ventricular dilatation. The walls appear echogenic. The cavity contains CSF and appears anechoic when seen.

- Corpus callosum:
  The corpus callosum is a midline structure that bridges horizontally to the roof of the lateral ventricles. It has an echogenic "double-walled"–like appearance. The parenchyma appears midgray or as medium- to low-level echoes.

- Cavum septum pellucidum and vergae:
  The cavum septum pellucidum (anterior portion) and vergae (posterior portion) appear comma-shaped sagitally or triangular-shaped coronally. This is a midline, anechoic, fluid-filled structure projecting superoanterior to the third ventricle and lies between the frontal horns and bodies of the two lateral ventricles.

- Thalamus:
  The two egg-shaped thalami lie on each side of the third ventricle. They appear midgray or as medium- to low-level echoes.

- Cerebellum:
  The cerebellum lies immediately posterior to the fourth ventricle and occupies the majority of the posterior fossae of the skull. The vermis is the central echogenic portion of the cerebellum, whereas the surrounding parenchyma appears midgray or as medium-level echoes.

- The cisterna magna:
  The cisterna magna is a small, anechoic, fluid-filled space, immediately postero-inferior to the cerebellum.

- Choroid plexus:
  The choroid plexus consists of two curvilinear, echogenic structures that arch around the thalami anteriorly from the floor of the body of the lateral ventricle and posteriorly to the tip of the temporal horn. Note that the choroid plexus does not extend into the frontal or occipital horns.

- Aqueduct of Sylvius:
  The aqueduct of Sylvius is a midline channel that connects the third and fourth ventricles. It is rarely seen sonographically unless dilated.

- Foramen of Monro:
  The foramen of Monro consists of anechoic, midline channels that connect the third ventricle with each lateral ventricle.

- Brain stem:
  The brain stem is a columnar-appearing structure that connects the forebrain and the spinal cord. Consists of the midbrain, pons, and the medulla oblongata. It appears midgray or as medium- to low-level echoes.

- Interhemispheric fissure:
  The interhemispheric fissure is a linear, echogenic area in which the midline falx lies separating the two cerebral hemispheres.

- Massa intermedia:
  The massa intermedia is a pea-shaped, soft tissue structure that is suspended within the third ventricle. It appears midgray or as medium-level echoes and is best seen with ventricular dilatation.

- Hippocampal gyrus (choroidal fissure):
  The hippocampal gyrus is an echogenic, spiral-like fold embodying each temporal horn.

- Cerebral peduncle:
  The cerebral peduncle is a medium- to low-level echo, Y-shaped structure inferior to the thalami and fused at the level of the pons.

- Sulci:
  The sulci are echogenic, spider-like fissures separating the gyri or folds of the brain. They appear fewer in number in the premature neonate.

- Tentorium:
  The tentorium is an echogenic structure (tent-shaped coronally) that separates the cerebrum from the inferior cerebellum and resembles a pine tree.

- Sylvian fissure:
  The sylvian fissure resembles an echogenic "Y" turned on its side and is located bilaterally between the temporal and frontal lobes of the brain. The middle cerebral artery can be seen pulsating here.

- Caudate nucleus:
  The caudate nucleus is located within the concavity of the lateral angles of each lateral ventricle and appears midgray or as medium-level echoes.

- Germinalmatrix/caudothalamicgroove:
  The germinal matrix is a vascular net-
  work located in the region of the caudate nucleus and thalamus called the
  caudothalamic groove. When visualized, it appears small and echogenic.
  Note that this is the most common site
  for a subependymal hemorrhage.

- Quadrigeminal plate:
  The quadrigeminal plate is an echogenic
  structure immediately superior to the
  apex of the tentorium resembling the
  top of a pine tree.

PATIENT PREP

- Keeping the infant warm is of utmost
  importance.

- The infant should be disturbed as little
  as possible, preferably left in the iso-
  lette.

- Gowns and gloves are recommended.

- The portable ultrasound system should
  be wiped down with a cleaning agent.

- Coupling gel should be body tempera-
  ture.

PATIENT POSITION

- Supine with the head face up.

- Prone with the head lying on either
  side.

TRANSDUCER

- 7.5 MHz. For premature infants less
  than 32 weeks' gestation or less than
  1500 g.

- 5.0 to 3.0 MHz for term and older infants
  with open anterior fontanelle.

NEONATAL BRAIN SURVEY

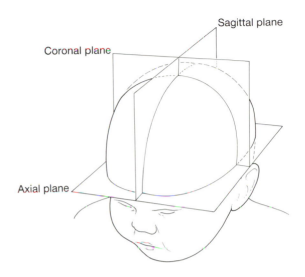

NOTE: Use the anterior fontanelle as a
window through which to angle or pivot
the transducer. The diameter of the fontanelle may restrict the amount of angu-
lation and anatomy seen.

NOTE: While surveying the brain, close
attention should be paid to all intracranial
anatomy and its symmetry.

CORONAL SURVEY

Coronal Plane/Anterior Fontanelle Approach

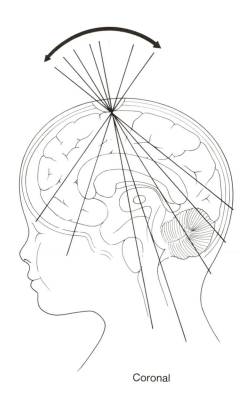

Coronal

- BEGIN WITH THE TRANSDUCER PER-PENDICULAR AT THE ANTERIOR FONTA-NELLE.
- SLOWLY ANGLE THE TRANSDUCER TO-WARD THE FACE. SCAN THROUGH THE FRONTAL HORNS INTO THE FRONTAL LOBES OF THE BRAIN.
- SLOWLY ANGLE THE TRANSDUCER BACK TO PERPENDICULAR.
- SLOWLY ANGLE THE TRANSDUCER POSTERIORLY. SCAN THROUGH THE OC-CIPITAL HORNS INTO THE OCCIPITAL LOBES OF THE BRAIN.
- SLOWLY ANGLE THE TRANSDUCER BACK TO PERPENDICULAR.

SAGITTAL SURVEY

Sagittal Plane/Anterior Fontanelle Approach

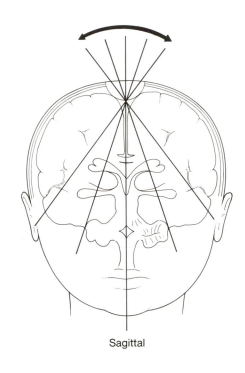

Sagittal

- BEGIN WITH THE TRANSDUCER PER-PENDICULAR AT THE ANTERIOR FONTA-NELLE.
- SLOWLY ANGLE THE TRANSDUCER LATERALLY TOWARD THE RIGHT LAT-ERAL VENTRICLE. SCAN THROUGH THE TEMPORAL LOBE OF THE BRAIN TO THE LEVEL OF THE SYLVIAN FISSURE.
- SLOWLY ANGLE THE TRANSDUCER BACK TO PERPENDICULAR.
- REPEAT THE FIRST, SECOND, AND THIRD STEPS, BUT ANGLE THE TRANS-DUCER THROUGH THE LEFT HEMI-SPHERE.

REQUIRED PICTURES

CORONAL IMAGES

Coronal Plane/Anterior Fontanelle Approach

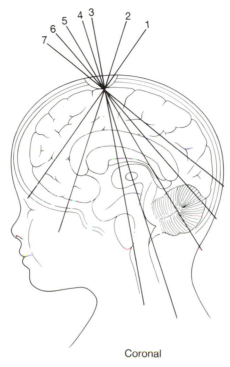

Coronal

1. CORONAL IMAGE OF THE FRONTAL LOBES OF THE BRAIN WITH THE IN-
TERHEMISPHERIC FISSURE. INCLUDE THE ORBITAL CONES AND ETH-
MOID SINUS.

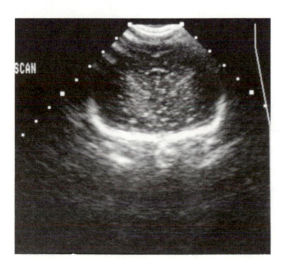

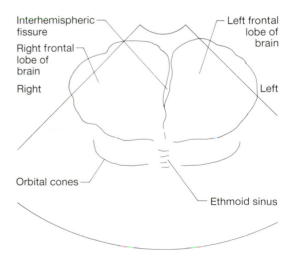

LABELED: CORONAL

2. CORONAL IMAGE OF THE FRONTAL HORNS OF THE VENTRICLES ENCOM-PASSING THE CAUDATE NUCLEUS. INCLUDE THE GERMINAL MATRIX ADJACENT TO THE VENTRICLES AND CORPUS CALLOSUM.

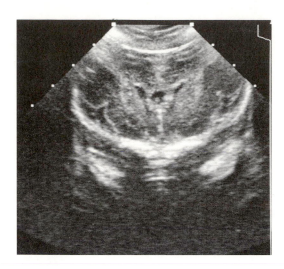 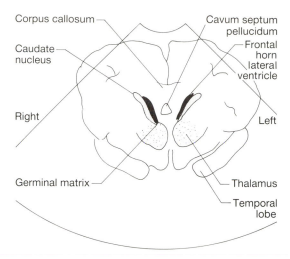

LABELED: CORONAL

3. CORONAL IMAGE OF THE FRONTAL HORNS AND THALAMI. INCLUDE THE SYLVIAN FISSURES, SEPTUM PELLUCIDUM, THIRD VENTRICLE, AND FO-RAMEN OF MONRO.

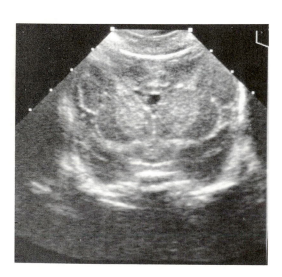 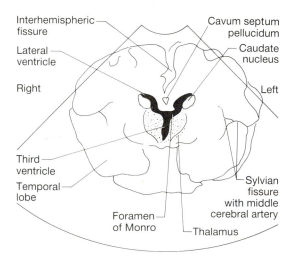

LABELED: CORONAL

4. CORONAL IMAGE OF THE BODIES OF THE LATERAL VENTRICLES, THAL-
   AMI, SYLVIAN FISSURES, CHOROIDAL FISSURES, AND TEMPORAL
   HORNS.

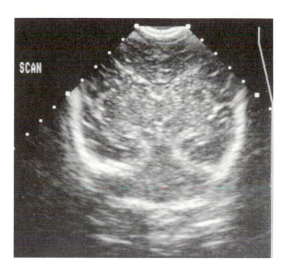

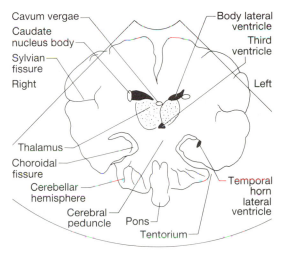

LABELED: CORONAL

5. CORONAL IMAGE OF THE TENTORIUM CEREBELLI. INCLUDE THE SYL-
   VIAN FISSURES AND THE CISTERNA MAGNA.

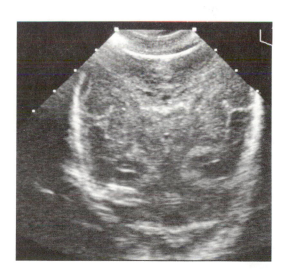

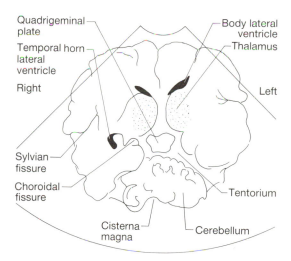

LABELED: CORONAL

6. CORONAL IMAGE OF THE CHOROID PLEXUS IN THE ATRIUM OR TRIGONE REGION.

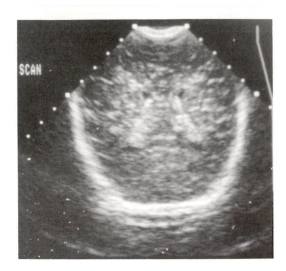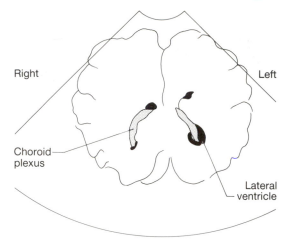

LABELED: CORONAL

7. CORONAL IMAGE OF THE OCCIPITAL LOBES OF THE BRAIN.

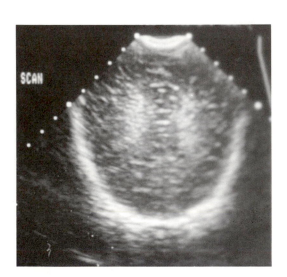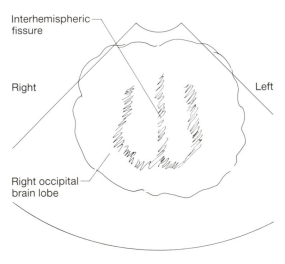

LABELED: CORONAL

SAGITTAL IMAGES

Sagittal Plane/Anterior Fontanelle Approach

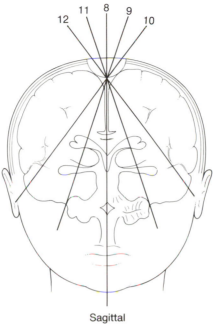

Sagittal

Midline Image

8. SAGITTAL MIDLINE IMAGE OF THE CAVUM SEPTUM PELLUCIDUM, COR-PUS CALLOSUM, THIRD VENTRICLE, FOURTH VENTRICLE, AND CERE-BELLUM, INCLUDING THE MASSA INTERMEDIA (SEEN IN TWO THIRDS OF INFANTS).

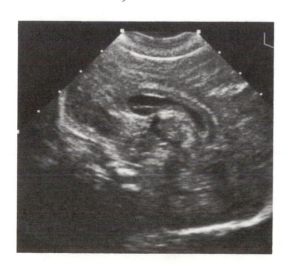
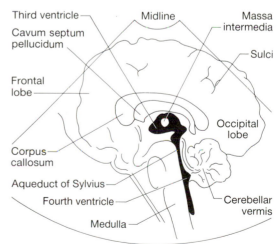

LABELED: SAG ML

NOTE: This image should be perpendicular at the midline.

Right Hemisphere Images

9. SAGITTAL IMAGE OF THE RIGHT VENTRICLE, GERMINAL MATRIX, CAUDATE NUCLEUS, THALAMUS, AND CHOROID PLEXUS.

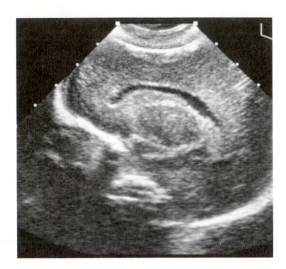
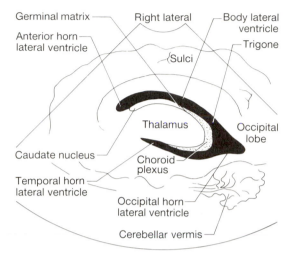

LABELED: SAG RT LAT

NOTE: In some cases the frontal horn, body, temporal horn, and occipital horn cannot be imaged in the same plane. Therefore an additional image(s) may be necessary. LABELED: **SAG RT LAT.**

10. SAGITTAL IMAGE OF THE RIGHT TEMPORAL LOBE OF THE BRAIN AT THE LEVEL OF THE SYLVIAN FISSURE.

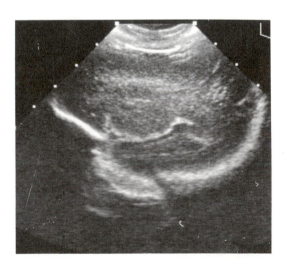
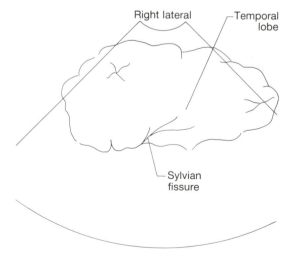

LABELED: SAG RT LAT

Left Hemisphere Images

11. SAGITTAL IMAGE OF THE LEFT VENTRICLE, GERMINAL MATRIX, CAU-
     DATE NUCLEUS, THALAMUS, AND CHOROID PLEXUS.

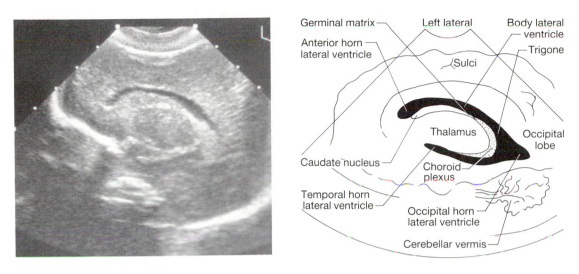

LABELED: SAG LT LAT

NOTE: In some cases the frontal horn, body, temporal horn, and occipital horn cannot
be imaged in the same plane. Therefore an additional image(s) may be necessary.
LABELED: **SAG LT LAT**

12. SAGITTAL IMAGE OF THE LEFT TEMPORAL LOBE OF THE BRAIN AT THE
     LEVEL OF THE SYLVIAN FISSURE.

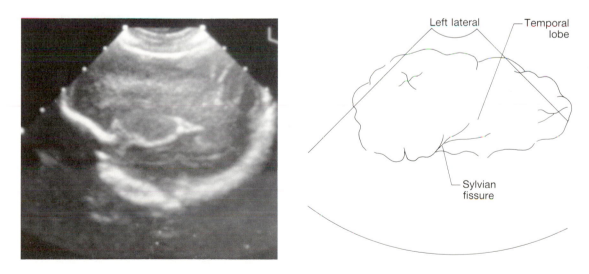

LABELED: SAG LT LAT

NOTE: Alternative axial views through the temporal recess or posterior fontanelle are
options to further evaluate the lateral ventricular walls and/or the occipital horns, respectively.

PART V

VASCULAR SCANNING PROTOCOLS

CHAPTER TWENTY-ONE
ABDOMINAL DOPPLER AND COLOR FLOW

FELICIA M. TERRY

BASIC PRINCIPLES

THE DOPPLER EQUATION

$$Fd = \frac{2\ Fo\ V\ COS\ \theta}{C}$$

Fd = Doppler frequency
Fo = Incident frequency
V = Flow velocity
C = Speed of sound
COS θ = Doppler angle

- As a sound beam is sent out into the body, any motion detected in the path of the beam is depicted as a change in frequency.

  - This is referred to as the Doppler shift frequency.

  - The Doppler shift frequency (Fd) increases as the operating frequency (Fo) increases.

  - The Doppler shift frequency usually falls within the audible frequency range.

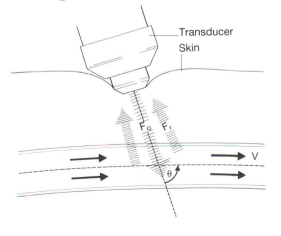

GENERAL INFORMATION

Frequency Range

- The diagnostic frequency range for ultrasound is 2 to 15 MHz.
  The frequency of choice depends on the depth of penetration required and the necessary resolution.

- As you increase the frequency you decrease depth of penetration, increase resolution, and increase blood flow detection.

Obtaining a Doppler signal from a moving target.

Angle Detection

- If quantitative information is needed, the Doppler angle must be known.

- The Doppler shift decreases as the doppler angle increases.

- This is usually operator-controllable and should be set between 45 and 60 degrees to ensure maximum signal return.

- If the Doppler angle select is set at 0 degrees, or parallel to flow, there will be no reflection of sound and therefore no returned Doppler signal.

- If the angle select is set at 90 degrees or perpendicular to flow, the computer will be unable to detect forward from reverse flow.

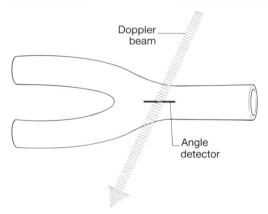

Image demonstrating proper Doppler angle correction. (Courtesy of Diasonics, Inc., Milpitas, California.)

Cursor Size

- When examining very small abdominal vessels, cursor size should be kept large to ensure that all vessel returns are detected.

- When examining larger vessels, the cursor size should be kept smaller.

  - Sampling should be complete throughout the entire vessel, but peak velocities are most likely to be encountered midvessel, and velocity samples taken for calculations should be taken midvessel.

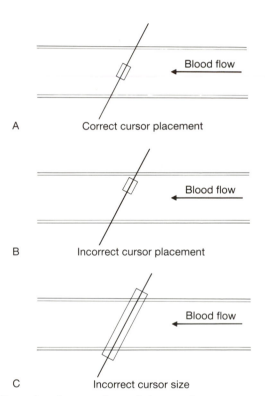

Examples of cursor size and placement.

Doppler Gains

- All gains should be set optimally to ensure proper window display without aliasing.

Common Doppler Controls

- Overall Doppler gain: will increase or decrease the total gain applied to the spectral Doppler image.

- Wall filter: will increase or decrease the echoes present because of wall "thumping." Must be careful not to set too high or you will wipe out useful information.

- Angle control: as discussed previously.

- Baseline: the scale may be changed to increase displayed velocity by adjusting this.

- Scale size: if operator-controllable, this can help eliminate aliasing when scanning with pulsed Doppler.

DOPPLER INSTRUMENTATION

Continuous Wave Doppler (CW)

- Cheaper.

- Generally a small pencil probe.

- Lacks axial resolution.

  - Cannot determine vessel depth.

  - Filters may be used to help decrease noise interference.

- An area of overlap between the outgoing and incoming beams is used as a basis for comparison to determine Doppler shift frequency.

  - A demodulator (often a quadrature phase detector) is used to determine the Doppler shift frequency.

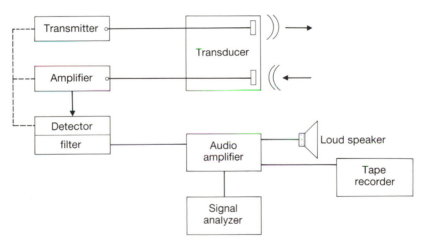

Block diagram of a continuous-wave Doppler system.

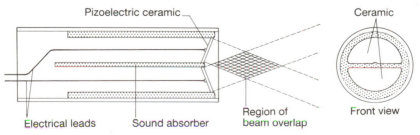

Diagram of a continuous-wave Doppler transducer.

Pulsed Wave Doppler (PW)

- Often duplex instrumentation. A combination of Doppler and real time instrumentation.

  - The Doppler image is superimposed over a Gray scale image.

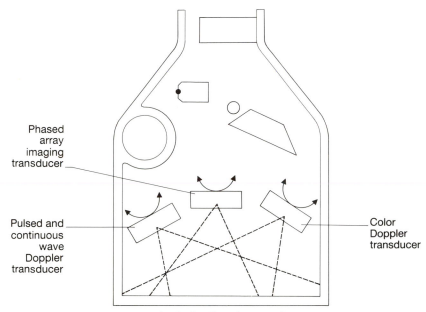

Phased array imaging transducer

Pulsed and continuous wave Doppler transducer

Color Doppler transducer

Diagram of a duplex Doppler transducer.

- The Doppler crystals are located within the imaging transducer.

- Allows Doppler analysis (temporal display) from a small, specific operator-controllable region.

- Is able to examine only a limited frequency range.

  - Will alias because the Doppler shift frequencies are determined through the use of multiple samples, and the internal computer may not be able to sample enough times because of time limitations (PRF).

- Has poor signal to noise ratios (it may be difficult to detect low flow signals because of noise interference).

  – Hard to remove noise without removing real information.

- May use high power levels:

  – SPTA levels may reach 1 W/cm^2

- The use of an operator-set Doppler angle correction allows easy calculation of flow velocities by the internal computer using the Doppler equation.

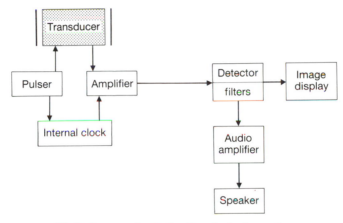

Block diagram of a duplex Doppler instrument.

Color Doppler

- Newer, more expensive technology.

- Offers a display of mean flow velocities (spatially) by sampling multiple points at a very fast rate.

- Multiple sampling often causes noise from tissue movement as well as from moving blood signals. Filters must be used to eliminate all but the continuously moving signals.

- Frequency shifts are detected through autocorrelation.

DOPPLER ANALYSIS

Audible Sound

- The Doppler shift frequency falls within the audible range of 200 Hz to 15 kHz.

Spectral Analysis

- The Doppler signal is displayed such that the power or intensity of each velocity is displayed as a shade of gray.

Color Doppler Analysis

- The color used for display is based on three characteristics of color.

  - Hue: the three primary colors are used to create color maps (red, blue, and green).

  - Saturation: the amount of white present in a color. This creates color shades.

  - Luminosity: the brightness of a color.

- Color Doppler systems typically use two monitors: one color and one Gray scale. There is better Gray scale resolution available on a dedicated Gray scale monitor because of increased spatial resolution.
  Larger color monitors allow better spatial resolution.

- Red flow generally represents flow toward the transducer.

- Blue flow generally represents flow away from the transducer.

- Yellow, white, or mosaic patterns represent high velocity or complex flow patterns.

- With color imaging, spectral broadening may be viewed as "variance."

  - One color is arbitrarily chosen to display a wide range of velocities present.

  - This color is often green.

- These patterns are operator-controllable.

- Other color Doppler controls:

  - The number of cycles per color line (often referred to as dwell time, ensemble length, or packet size).
    If this is increased, flow sensitivity increases, but frame rate decreases.

  - Gray scale/color priority: This determines whether Gray scale or color Doppler information will be emphasized in display.
    Increasing this increases the color saturation.
    Decreasing this helps to decrease the color present from wall and tissue motion.
    This acts as a filter by suppressing color information above a certain operator-set level.

DOPPLER PITFALLS

Aliasing

- Does not occur with CW Doppler.

- Occurs in PW and color Doppler at the **Nyquist limit.**

- The maximum frequency level that can be displayed is equal to one half of the system's PRF (pulse repetition frequency). If the Doppler frequency exceeds that level, aliasing will occur.

- Appearance: An aliased signal will wrap around the baseline or may appear as concurrent reversed flow.

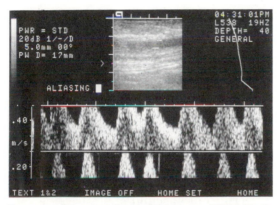

Example of Doppler aliasing. (Courtesy of Mary Washington Hospital, Fredericksburg, Virginia.)

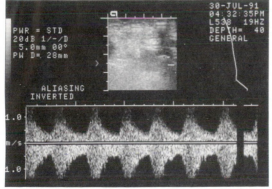

Example of Doppler aliasing. (Courtesy of Mary Washington Hospital, Fredericksburg, Virginia.)

- This phenomenon occurs because the pulsed Doppler system cannot sample quickly enough.

- Aliasing may also occur in color Doppler systems.
  It will appear as an abrupt color change within the same vessel that is not caused by flow reversal.
  It is often seen as a change in high-frequency color codes (i.e., light red to light blue).

- Flow reversal will be seen as adjacent deep shades on the color map.

- Since red blood cells cause Rayleigh scattering, and as you increase frequency you increase Rayleigh scattering, we must, just as in Gray scale imaging, find the incident frequency that gives adequate penetration with acceptable resolution and signal amplitude without aliasing.

Color Imaging Pitfalls

NOTE: Like PW Doppler, color Doppler is limited by the frame rate, tissue depth, and PRF of the system.

- Color Doppler systems tend to have poorer resolution.

- Color Doppler systems are unable to detect flow less than approximately 0.05 meters per second.

  - If there is a low-flow color map available, color may well be the best way to visualize low-velocity flow because with CW or PW Doppler, low-flow signals are often covered up by noise or eliminated by the wall filter (set too high).

  - Color Doppler systems use frame rates of 4 to 32 frames per second.

  - This may be operator-controllable. Increase for better resolution.

  - To better detect low-velocity flow use a higher frequency transducer.

  - To decrease the tissue or vessel wall vibrations, decrease the color wall filter.

- Mirror image artifacts:
  - To correct range ambiguity artifacts:
    - Decrease PRF.
    - Increase frequency of the transducer.
    - Decrease far gain.
  - Grating lobes:
    - Result from decreased lateral resolution because the beam is not perpendicular to the target.
    - To correct, adjust the transducer angle and/or Doppler steering angle.

BIOLOGICAL EFFECTS

- The American Institute of Ultrasound in Medicine states that for imaging transducers no known bioeffects have been proved below scanning intensity levels of 100 mW/cm^2 SPTA.

- No known bioeffects have been documented at currently used diagnostic intensity levels.

- All sonographers should be familiar with their equipment and the intensity levels stated by the manufacturer's owner's manual.

- All sonographers should scan conscientiously at all times.

- The AIUM recommends scanning on a "when needed" basis. This practice ensures that the valuable information we produce diagnostically will continue to outweigh any remote risk that may exist.

- The AIUM has approved fetal Doppler for the examination of the fetal heart and umbilical cord.

PURPOSE OF ABDOMINAL DOPPLER AND/OR COLOR FLOW DOPPLER

- To determine vascular versus avascular nature of abdominal masses.
- To assess anomalous vessels.
- To confirm normal anatomy.
- To determine vessel pulsatility.
- To determine the amount of flow resistance present.
  - Cirrhotic liver disease.
  - Renal transplants.
  - Assessment of high-risk pregnancy.
  - Formulae used:

Resistive index:
$$\frac{A - B}{A} \qquad (1)$$

Pulsatility index:
$$\frac{\text{Peak Systolic V} - \text{End Diastolic V}}{\text{Mean Velocity}} \qquad (2)$$

- To rule out vascular stenosis.
- To rule out vessel thrombosis.
- To determine flow rates.
- To determine flow direction.
- To assess shunt detection.
  - To determine shunt patency in Budd-Chiari syndrome patients.

CLINICAL NOTES

EXAMINATION PROTOCOL

- Abdominal Doppler and/or color flow is rarely if ever done as an examination in and of itself. It is usually done in conjunction with a full abdominal examination to add additional information to the gray scale images.

ARTERIAL FLOW

- Pulsates with cardiac cycle.
- Most arterial flow within the abdomen has fairly low resistance.

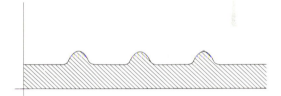

Example of a low-resistance arterial signal.

- This typically means that the signal will not cross the baseline.
- Low flow vessels or abdominal masses often have a spectral appearance with lower systolic peaks and a more pronounced diastolic component.

● Examples of abdominal arterial flow.

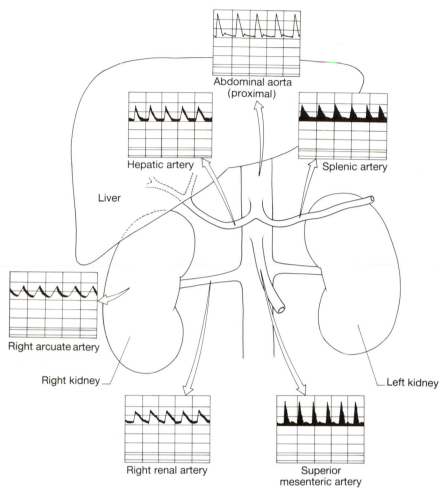

Examples of abdominal arterial flow signals.

NOTE: Each vessel has a characteristic appearance.

The investigation of certain vessels may add valuable information to the clinical question concerning the presence of pathology.

- Hepatic arteries:
  Tend to have low impedance flow with a high diastolic component.
  Need to confirm the presence of flow for liver transplants.
  Increased flow may indicate portal hypertension or portal vein thrombosis.

- Superior mesenteric artery: see section on mesenteric ischemia.

- Renal arteries:
  Assess renal artery stenosis caused by hypertension or decreased renal function.
  Normal resistance: peak systolic velocities <100 cm/second. Persistent decreasing diastolic flow due to low resistance.
  Mild resistance to moderate resistance: decreased diastolic flow component. Slower systolic peaking.
  Severe resistance: peak systolic velocities >1 meter/second. Increased ratio of renal to aortic peak systolic velocities (>3.5). Increased turbulence due to increased impedance. At worst, no detectable flow.

- Renal transplants:
  Rejection: Often see decreased blood flow due to decreased renal function and increased capillary resistance (often due to external compression or narrowing of smaller blood vessels). There will be decreased diastolic flow.
  Infarction: helps to detect even very low flow states.
  Renal artery stenosis: as discussed previously.

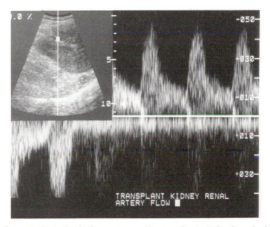

Spectral analysis from a renal transplant at the level of the renal artery. (Courtesy of Mary Washington Hospital, Fredericksburg, Virginia.)

- Miscellaneous:
  Blood supply to any area of interest.

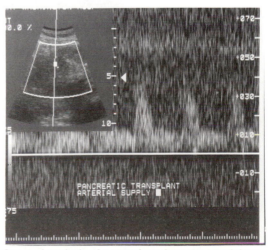

Spectral analysis of a waveform from the arterial supply to a pancreatic transplant. (Courtesy of Mary Washington Hospital, Fredericksburg, Virginia.)

● Arterial color Doppler of the abdomen:

  – Select images:
    Renal arteries.
    Renal profusion.
    Hepatic artery at porta hepatis.

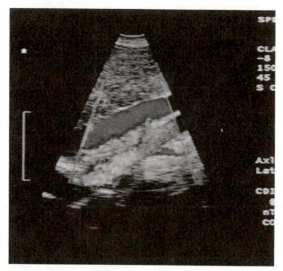

Color Doppler image demonstrating renal artery origins. See Color Plate 1 at the back of this book. (Courtesy of Diasonics, Inc., Milpitas, California.)

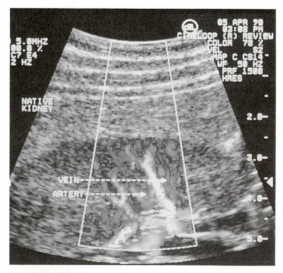

Color Doppler image demonstrating renal perfusion. See Color Plate 2 at the back of this book. (Courtesy of ATL, Bothell, Washington.)

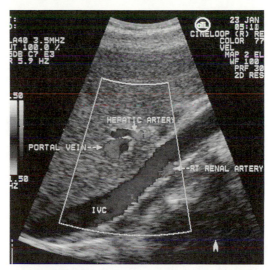

Color Doppler image demonstrating flow in the region of the porta hepatis. See Color Plate 3 at the back of this book. (Courtesy of ATL, Bothell, Washington.)

VENOUS FLOW

- The amount of respiratory changes seen varies.

  - Portal veins and splenic veins show little or no respiratory variations.

  - In venous hypertension, the splanchnic vessels will dilate to diameters greater than 1.5 cm.

- Clinical examples:

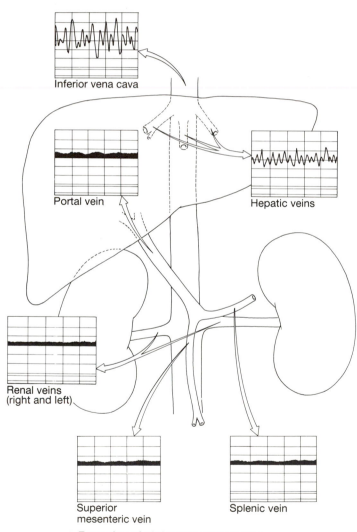

Inferior vena cava

Portal vein

Hepatic veins

Renal veins (right and left)

Superior mesenteric vein

Splenic vein

Examples of abdominal venous flow signals.

● Clinical notes:

– Inferior vena cava:
Must document patent flow for liver transplants.
Rule out thrombosis invasion by renal masses.
To assess thrombosis surrounding IVC clips or filters.

– Splenic vein: see section on mesenteric ischemia.

– Portal vein:
Normally has steady flow.
The presence of respiratory variations (biphasic signals) suggests portal hypertension. This is due to increased resistance.
Differentiation of portal vein branches from dilated biliary ducts.

– Renal veins:
Determine the presence of thrombosis:
May vary in echogenicity.
May cause an increase in vein size.
Differentiation of renal vein from hydronephrosis.

● Venous color Doppler of the abdomen.

– Hepatic veins.

– Portal vein.

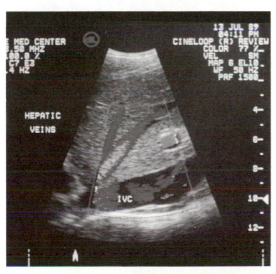

Example of color flow Doppler in hepatic veins. See Color Plate 4 at the back of this book. (Courtesy of ATL, Bothell, Washington.)

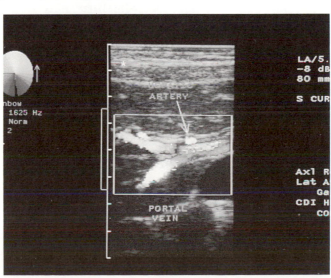

Example of color Doppler image of flow in the portal vein. See Color Plate 5 at the back of this book. (Courtesy of Diasonics, Inc., Milpitas, California.)

MISCELLANEOUS

- Vascular tumors: often have three primary characteristics:

  - High-amplitude signals.

  - Increased peak systolic velocities.

  - A "roaring" sound due to edge motion and interference from the increased vascularity.

- Hepatomata: Demonstrate high pitched signals due to arteriovenous communications.

- Pseudoaneurysm: May have disorganized, pulsatile, or circular flow with low-velocity signals in a hypo- or anechoic mass.
  These are most often near a vessel anastomosis.
  If fully clotted, there will be no flow present.

- A/V fistulae (arteriovenous fistulae).

  - The arterial component will show increased flow velocities with decreased resistive index.

  - The venous component will show increased pulsatility.

- Mesenteric ischemia.

  - Turbulent arterial signals.

  - Retrograde venous flow in the splenic vein.

  - After a meal is given, a normal patient should show the following superior mesenteric artery flow changes:
    Increased flow.
    Decreased diastolic flow reversal.
    Increased diastolic forward flow.

  - With mesenteric ischemia, after a meal no flow changes occur.

- Gallbladder cancer versus sludge.

  - A cancer will show some low flow.

  - Sludge shows no flow.

GYNECOLOGICAL STUDIES

- An active ovary shows increased peak systolic flow and a diastolic flow component.

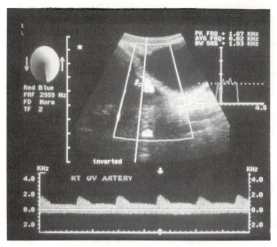

Doppler spectral display of blood flow in an active ovary. (Courtesy of Diasonics, Inc., Milpitas, California.)

- An inactive ovary shows no diastolic flow component.

  - Diastolic flow decreases normally during the follicular phase of ovulation.

- Ectopic pregnancies: spectral or color Doppler may help to show trophoblastic flow with high diastolic flow components.

- Infertility: may help to determine the presence of ovarian flow of ovulation.

OBSTETRICAL STUDIES

N O T E : Remember to scan prudently.

- The flow resistance within the umbilical artery may be directly related to the presence of intrauterine growth retardation.
  The umbilical artery may show the following changes when IUGR is present due to increased placental pressure: Increased resistance.
  Decreased diastolic flow in the umbilical artery.

- Doppler of the umbilical cord:
  - To identify a three-vessel cord.
  - To assess cord insertions.
  - To rule out nuchal cord.

- Doppler of the fetal heart; will help to identify cardiac chambers and flow patterns.

- Doppler of the placenta.
  - Rule out chorioangiomata versus placental lakes.

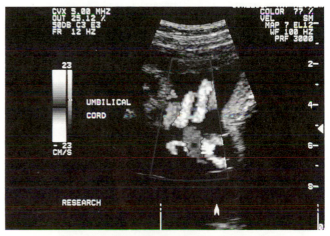

Color Doppler image of a three-vessel umbilical cord. See Color Plate 6 at the back of this book. (Courtesy of ATL, Bothell, Washington.)

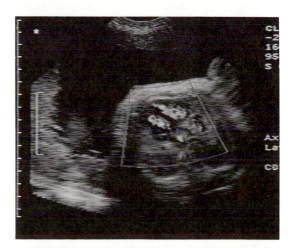

Color Doppler image of a fetal four-chamber heart. See Color Plate 7 at the back of this book. (Courtesy of Diasonics, Inc., Milpitas, California. Diasonics does not have the Food and Drug Administration approval to market their probes for this fetal Doppler application. However, the final decision as to how a medical device will be used is the prerogative of the medical practitioner. Please check FDA approval for all manufacturers' probes used in any examination.)

BREAST SONOGRAPHY

- Current studies are showing an increase in detection of Doppler signals in malignant lesions versus nonmalignant lesions.

SCROTAL ULTRASOUND

- The testicular artery has low peripheral resistance with broad systolic peaks and high diastolic flow.

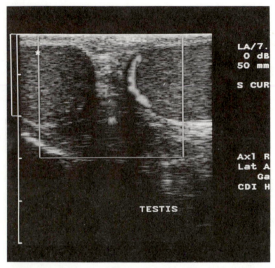

Color Doppler image demonstrating arterial flow in a testicular artery. See Color Plate 8 at the back of this book. (Courtesy of Diasonics, Inc., Milpitas, California.)

- The deferential artery has high resistance with narrow systolic peaks and low diastolic flow.

- Pathology:

  - Inflammatory conditions:
    Epididymitis.
    Orchitis.
    Abscesses:
    Demonstrate hypervascularity.
    Have decreased RI indices.
    Gray scale shows decreased echogenicity due to swelling.

  - Torsion/ischemia:
    Complete or near complete absence of flow.
    Nuclear medicine is still the study of choice.

  - Neoplasms:
    Gray scale images remain most helpful in defining masses.
    Doppler or color Doppler may help define vascular tumors.

  - Varicoceles:
    These are often easily visible.
    A vein greater than 3 mm during a Valsalva maneuver is considered a varicocele.

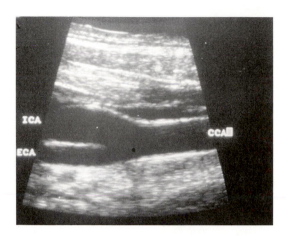

Longitudinal image of the carotid artery bifurcation.
(Courtesy of Diasonics, Inc., Milpitas, California.)

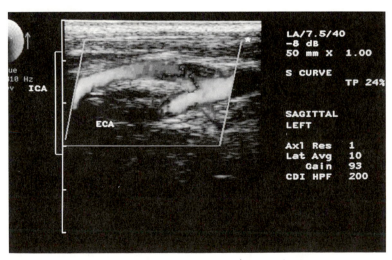

Color Doppler image of the carotid artery bifurcation. (See Color Plate 9 at the back of this book.) (Courtesy of Diasonics, Inc., Milpitas, California.)

CHAPTER TWENTY-TWO
DUPLEX CAROTID ARTERY SCANNING PROTOCOL

FELICIA M. TERRY

LOCATION

- Medial to internal jugular vein.

- Lateral to thyroid gland.

- Posteromedial to the sternocleidomas-toid muscle.

ANATOMY

- Right common carotid artery originates off of the innominate artery.

- Left common carotid artery originates off of the aortic arch.

- At approximately the level of the thy-roid cartilage, the common carotid ar-tery bifurcates into a more anterome-dial external carotid artery and a more posterolateral internal carotid artery.

- The external carotid artery can be dif-ferentiated from the internal carotid ar-tery by looking for branches within the neck.

- The internal carotid artery tends to be larger than the external, although size is variable.

PHYSIOLOGY

- The external carotid artery provides vascular flow to the face and facial muscles.

- The internal carotid artery provides vascular flow to the internal brain structures.

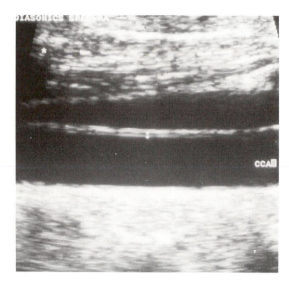

Common carotid artery. (Courtesy of Diasonics, Inc., Milpitas, California.)

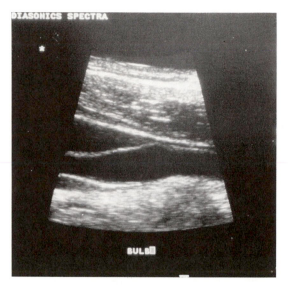

Carotid artery bulb. (Courtesy of Diasonics, Inc., Milpitas, California.)

Sonographic Appearance

- The internal vessel should be echo-free.

- If viewing the vessel at a perpendicular angle, you may be able to appreciate the intimal lining.

- You should be able to view the common, internal, and external carotid arteries as separate.

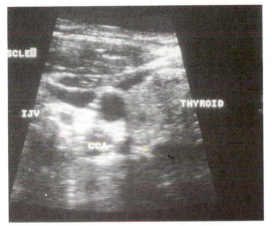

Common carotid artery. Note the sternocleidomastoid muscle. (Courtesy of Diasonics, Inc., Milpitas, California.)

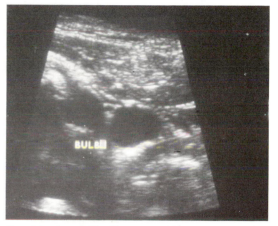

Carotid artery bulb. (Courtesy of Diasonics, Inc., Milpitas, California.)

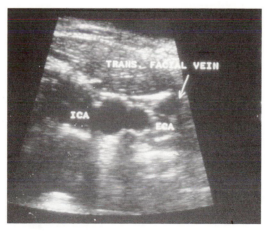

Internal and external carotid artery origins. (Courtesy of Diasonics, Inc., Milpitas, California.)

PATIENT PREP

- None.

PATIENT POSITION

- Supine with the neck slightly hyperextended using a rolled towel or small pillow to help extend neck.

- You may sit at the head of the table with the patient's head directly in front of you and able to rest your elbow on the corner of the table. You must then scan ambidextrously to be easily able to reach the machine.

- Or you may stand next to the patient table and lean one arm across the patient's chest in order to reach the neck. A pillow may be placed over the patient's chest in order to ensure patient comfort.

- The examination may be performed with the patient in an erect position if unable to lie down.

TRANSDUCER

- 10 MHz—better resolution, may not be able to visualize all anatomy if vessels lie deep within the neck.

- 7.5 MHz—allows slightly better penetration.

- 5.0 MHz—with a standoff pad—greatly reduces resolution.

SURVEY

- BEGIN IN ANTERIOR, CORONAL (LATERAL), OR POSTERIOR SCANNING PLANE.
- START ON THE RIGHT SIDE IMMEDIATELY SUPERIOR TO THE CLAVICLE. MOVE LATERAL AND IDENTIFY THE JUGULAR VEIN. MOVE MEDIALLY THROUGH THE COMMON CAROTID ARTERY AND IDENTIFY THE THYROID GLAND.
- RETURN TO A LONGITUDINAL VIEW OF THE COMMON CAROTID ARTERY AND ANGLE AS INFERIORLY AS POSSIBLE IN ORDER TO VIEW AS MUCH OF THE ORIGIN AS POSSIBLE.
- MOVE SUPERIORLY, CONTINUOUSLY ROCKING THROUGH THE VESSEL MEDIAL TO LATERAL IN ORDER TO VIEW AS MUCH OF THE VESSEL WALLS AS POSSIBLE.
- WHILE AT THE LEVEL OF THE MIDDLE COMMON CAROTID ARTERY, ANGLE THE PROBE IN A POSTEROLATERAL MANNER AND LOOK FOR THE VERTEBRAL BODIES. RUNNING IN BETWEEN THE VERTEBRAL BODIES YOU SHOULD SEE THE VERTEBRAL ARTERY, WHICH OFTEN LIES POSTERIOR TO THE VERTEBRAL VEIN. ANGLE THE PROBE IN A VERY SLIGHTLY MEDIAL/LATERAL MANNER TO ENSURE THE BEST VISUALIZATION OF THE ARTERY.

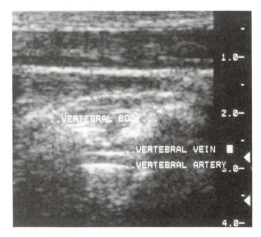

Vertebral artery. (Courtesy of Mary Washington Hospital, Fredericksburg, Virginia.)

• ANGLE THE PROBE ANTEROMEDIAL AND RETURN TO THE COMMON CAROTID SURVEY.

• CONTINUE SUPERIORLY TO THE LEVEL OF THE BIFURCATION, THEN ROCK IN AN ANTEROMEDIAL/POSTEROLATERAL MOTION AND IDENTIFY BOTH THE INTERNAL AND EXTERNAL CAROTID ARTERIES.

• CONTINUE TO MOVE SUPERIORLY WITH A SLIGHTL POSTEROMEDIAL ANGLE TO VIEW THE INTERNAL CAROTID ARTERY. CONTINUE TO ROCK LATERAL TO MEDIAL TO VIEW THE VESSEL WALLS COMPLETELY. FOLLOW THE VESSEL AS SUPERIORLY AS POSSIBLE TO THE MANDIBLE.

NOTE: As you move superiorly, it may be easier to view a greater length of the internal carotid artery by moving from a more anterior or lateral approach to a more posterior approach.

• RETURN INFERIORLY TO THE LEVEL OF THE BULB AND ROCK ANTEROMEDIALLY TO IDENTIFY THE EXTERNAL CAROTID ARTERY. MOVE SUPERIORLY ALONG THE LENGTH OF THE EXTERNAL CAROTID ARTERY ROCKING LATERAL AND MEDIALLY THROUGH THE VESSEL TO FULLY VISUALIZE WALLS.

NOTE: Follow each vessel as superiorly as possible until the mandible makes it impossible to go further.

• ONCE YOU HAVE VIEWED BOTH THE INTERNAL AND EXTERNAL CAROTID ARTERIES IN A LONGITUDINAL PLANE, MOVE INFERIORLY AGAIN BACK TO THE LEVEL IMMEDIATELY SUPERIOR TO THE CLAVICLE.

• ROTATE THE TRANSDUCER 90 DEGREES AND BEGIN THE TRANSVERSE SURVEY ON THE RIGHT COMMON CAROTID ARTERY.

• ANGLE AS INFERIORLY AS POSSIBLE NOTING AS MUCH OF THE ORIGIN AS POSSIBLE. IT MAY BE POSSIBLE TO VIEW THE SUBCLAVIAN ARTERY AT THIS LEVEL.

• MOVE SUPERIORLY NOTING VESSEL WALLS AND INTERNAL COMPONENTS.

• MAKE SPECIAL NOTE OF THE BIFURCATION AND VIEW THE INTERNAL AND EXTERNAL CAROTID ARTERIES SUPERIORLY TO THE BIFURCATION.

• FOLLOW AS SUPERIORLY AS POSSIBLE TO THE MANDIBLE.

• MOVE INFERIORLY AGAIN TO THE LEVEL OF THE CLAVICLE. ROTATE THE PROBE 90 DEGREES AND BEGIN THE SPECTRAL SURVEY BY TURNING ON THE DOPPLER SAMPLE VOLUME (REFER TO OWNER'S MANUAL FOR EQUIPMENT SPECIFICATIONS). FOLLOW THE VESSEL LONGITUDINALLY, ADJUSTING THE SAMPLE VOLUME TO MAINTAIN A MIDVESSEL LOCATION.

• BE SURE TO SAMPLE ADEQUATELY THROUGHOUT THE BULB AREA AND THROUGH EACH OF THE INTERNAL AND EXTERNAL CAROTID ARTERIES.

• WITH THE SAMPLE VOLUME STILL ON, MOVE INFERIORLY BACK TO A LEVEL IMMEDIATELY SUPERIOR TO THE CLAVICLE. THIS ACTS AS A SECOND SAMPLING AND ENSURES A COMPLETE DOPPLER INVESTIGATION. NOW MOVE TOWARD THE LEVEL OF THE MIDDLE COMMON CAROTID, AND ANGLING THE PROBE POSTEROLATERAL, SAMPLE THE VERTEBRAL ARTERY.

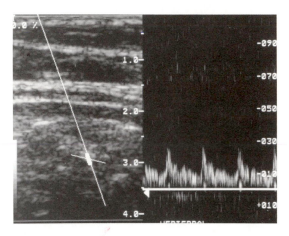

Spectral display of vertebral artery blood flow. (Courtesy of Mary Washington Hospital, Fredericksburg, Virginia.)

NOTE: If plaquing is present, be sure to sample all around checking for hemodynamic significance.

• ONCE FLOW HAS BEEN ASSESSED THOROUGHLY IN ALL VESSELS, YOU MAY RETURN TO THE COMMON CAROTID ARTERY AND BEGIN TO OBTAIN THE REQUIRED IMAGES.

NOTE: Deep vessel bifurcation may make it very hard to differentiate vessels by appearance alone. Always use Doppler signals.

NOTE: Long-standing occlusions of the internal carotid artery may cause an enlargement of the external carotid artery and its branches, which may cuase erroneous vessel identification.

NOTE: Normal vessel turbulence is possible and should not be mistaken for pathology. Look for vessel bends or kinks.

NOTE: When scanning with color Doppler it is easiest to turn the color Doppler on after the longitudinal and transverse gray scale survey.

• ONCE THE TRANSVERSE SURVEY HAS BEEN COMPLETED, RETURN TO THE LEVEL OF THE CLAVICLE AND TURN ON THE COLOR DOPPLER. SET COLOR GAINS, AND SO FORTH. THE STEERING ANGLE WILL BE KEPT PERPENDICULAR.
• THEN PERFORM A TRANSVERSE SURVEY IN THE SAME MANNER AS YOU WOULD A GRAY SCALE SURVEY PASS. YOU MAY NEED TO SCAN MORE SLOWLY TO ALLOW PROPER COLOR FILLING OF THE VESSEL LUMEN.

● WHEN YOU HAVE SCANNED AS SUPERIORLY AS POSSIBLE, AGAIN RETURN TO THE LEVEL OF THE CLAVICLE. ROTATE THE PROBE 90 DEGREES AND ADJUST THE COLOR DOPPLER STEERING ANGLE ACCORDING TO THE LIE OF THE VESSEL. FOLLOW THE VESSEL SUPERIORLY. IT IS OFTEN NECESSARY TO CHANGE THE STEERING ANGLE AT LEAST ONCE AS THE VESSEL CHANGES LIE. THE STEERING ANGLE SHOULD REMAIN AS CLOSE TO PARALLEL TO THE ANGLE OF FLOW AS POSSIBLE.

● ONCE THE COMMON, INTERNAL, AND EXTERNAL CAROTID VESSELS HAVE BEEN THOROUGHLY INVESTIGATED, YOU MAY RETURN TO THE LEVEL OF THE MIDDLE COMMON CAROTID ARTERY, LOCATE THE VERTEBRAL ARTERY, AND CONFIRM FLOW.

● YOU MAY THEN RETURN TO THE LEVEL OF THE CLAVICLE AND BEGIN TO OBTAIN YOUR SPECTRAL TRACINGS.

● COLOR DOPPLER MAY BE LEFT ON FOR THE REMAINDER OF THE EXAMINATION, ALTHOUGH COLOR DOPPLER CANNOT REPLACE THE SPECTRAL ANALYSIS THROUGHOUT THE VESSEL. IT MAY, HOWEVER, HELP YOU TO IDENTIFY HIGH-VELOCITY JETS THROUGH WHICH YOU MAY WANT TO SAMPLE MORE CAREFULLY.

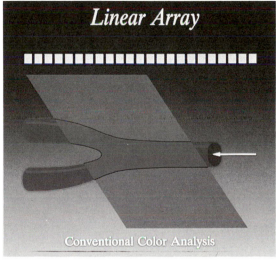

Color Doppler angle adjustment. (Courtesy of Diasonics, Inc., Milpitas, California.)

REQUIRED PICTURES

1. LONGITUDINAL IMAGE OF THE RIGHT PROXIMAL COMMON CAROTID ARTERY.

    LABELED: LONG (OR SAG) RT PCCA

2. SPECTRAL ANALYSIS IMAGE OF WAVEFORM FROM THE RIGHT PROXIMAL COMMON CAROTID ARTERY WITH PEAK SYSTOLIC AND END DIASTOLIC VELOCITIES MEASURED.

    LABELED: RT PCCA

3. LONGITUDINAL IMAGE OF THE RIGHT DISTAL COMMON CAROTID ARTERY.

    LABELED: LONG (OR SAG) RT DCCA

4. SPECTRAL ANALYSIS OF WAVEFORM FROM THE RIGHT DISTAL COMMON CAROTID ARTERY WITH PEAK SYSTOLIC AND END DIASTOLIC VELOCITIES MEASURED.

    LABELED: RT DCCA

5. LONGITUDINAL IMAGE OF THE RIGHT PROXIMAL INTERNAL CAROTID ARTERY SHOWING ITS ORIGIN FROM THE BULB.

    LABELED: LONG (OR SAG) RT PICA

6. SPECTRAL ANALYSIS IMAGE OF WAVEFORM FROM THE PROXIMAL INTERNAL CAROTID ARTERY WITH PEAK SYSTOLIC AND END DIASTOLIC VELOCITIES MEASURED.

    LABELED: DIST RT ICA

7. LONGITUDINAL IMAGE OF THE RIGHT MIDDLE INTERNAL CAROTID ARTERY.

    LABELED: LONG (OR SAG) RT MICA

8. SPECTRAL ANALYSIS IMAGE OF WAVEFORM FROM THE MIDDLE INTERNAL CAROTID ARTERY WITH PEAK SYSTOLIC AND END DIASTOLIC VELOCITIES MEASURED.

LABELED: RT MICA

9. LONGITUDINAL IMAGE OF THE RIGHT DISTAL INTERNAL CAROTID ARTERY.

LABELED: LONG (OR SAG) RT DICA

10. SPECTRAL ANALYSIS IMAGE OF WAVEFORM FROM THE DISTAL INTERNAL CAROTID ARTERY WITH PEAK SYSTOLIC AND END DIASTOLIC VELOCITIES MEASURED.

LABELED: RT DICA

11. LONGITUDINAL IMAGE OF THE RIGHT EXTERNAL CAROTID ARTERY.

LABELED: LONG (OR SAG) RT ECA

12. SPECTRAL ANALYSIS IMAGE OF WAVEFORM FROM THE EXTERNAL CAROTID ARTERY WITH PEAK SYSTOLIC AND END DIASTOLIC VELOCITIES MEASURED.

LABELED: RT ECA

13. OPTIONAL: LONGITUDINAL IMAGE OF THE RIGHT VERTEBRAL ARTERY.

LABELED: LONG (OR SAG) RT VERT

NOTE: The spectral image of this vessel is often not satisfactory because of the depth of the vertebral vessels.

14. SPECTRAL ANALYSIS IMAGE OF WAVEFORM FROM THE VERTEBRAL ARTERY WITH PEAK SYSTOLIC AND END DIASTOLIC VELOCITIES MEASURED.

LABELED: RT VERT

15. TRANSVERSE IMAGE OF THE CAROTID BULB JUST PRIOR TO VESSEL BIFURCATION.

LABELED: TRNS RT BULB

NOTE: Any stenosis present must be imaged and measured. Area/circumference measurements preferred. Even though stenosis will most commonly be seen at the carotid bulb, it is often found in other areas of the vessels. Stenosis at any level must be imaged transversely with and without area reduction measurements and labeled according to their location appropriately.

NOTE: Even when no disease is present, it is important to image the area of the bulb. This area is most prone to disease processes because of its natural turbulence. Stenotic lesions are often not symptomatic until they reach 60% lumen reduction or more and may be discovered only with careful scanning in the transverse plane.

NOTE: All stenotic plaque should be measured in the transverse plane to ensure the highest accuracy.

NOTE: Additional images of plaque may be necessary. It is important to look for irregularities along the borders of the plaque, which may indicate ulcerations.

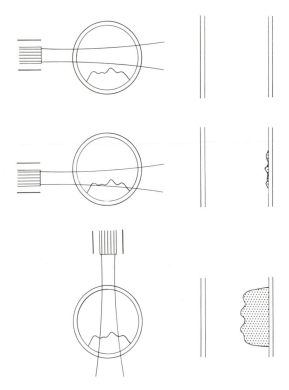

The importance of thoroughly examining the vessel is shown here. With an improper survey, this plaque might be missed.

Repeat on the left side beginning with a thorough survey and then continuing on to take the required images.

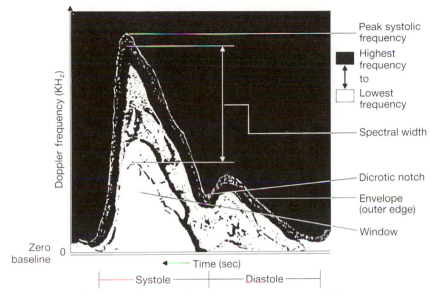

Example of a spectral display from the carotid arteries.

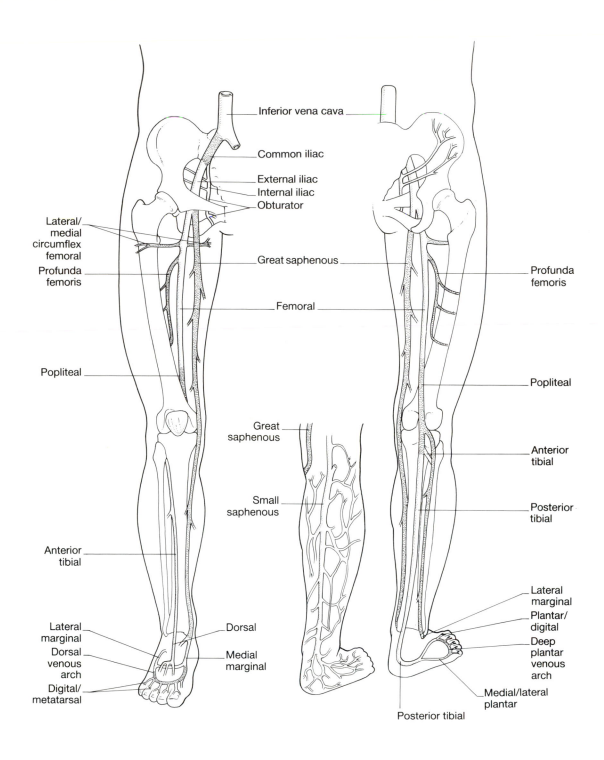

Inferior vena cava

Common iliac

External iliac

Internal iliac

Obturator

Lateral/
medial
circumflex
femoral

Profunda
femoris

Great saphenous

Profunda
femoris

Femoral

Popliteal

Popliteal

Great
saphenous

Anterior
tibial

Small
saphenous

Posterior
tibial

Anterior
tibial

Lateral
marginal

Dorsal

Plantar/
digital

Lateral
marginal

Dorsal
venous
arch

Medial
marginal

Deep
plantar
venous
arch

Digital/
metatarsal

Medial/lateral
plantar

Posterior tibial

VENOUS SYSTEM OF
THE LOWER LIMB

Normal deep and superficial venous anatomy of the legs.

CHAPTER TWENTY-THREE
PERIPHERAL VASCULAR
SCANNING PROTOCOLS

FELICIA M. TERRY

LOWER EXTREMITY VENOUS DUPLEX ULTRASONOGRAPHY

- Purpose: to noninvasively determine the presence of venous thrombosis.

ANATOMY

- The common femoral vein (CFV) lies medial to the common femoral artery (CFA).

- The superficial vein (SFV) lies posterior to the superficial femoral artery (SFA) superiorly.

- The SFV follows a medial course along the inner curve of the thigh and at its inferior aspect, just superior to the knee, lies posterior to the SFA.

- The popliteal vein lies posterior and lateral to the popliteal artery.

- The saphenous vein is located medial to the SFV and CFV at the level of the SFV insertion.

- Valves are commonly seen in the larger veins to prevent the back flow of blood. These are often seen in the CFV, SFV, and sometimes in the popliteal veins.

- The deep femoral vein or profunda vein is found posterior to the SFV with its insertion at approximately the same level.

- All veins are thin-walled and collapse easily with a minimum of pressure.

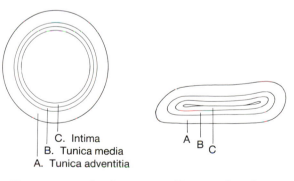

C. Intima
B. Tunica media
A. Tunica adventitia

Noncompressed and compressed images of a vein.

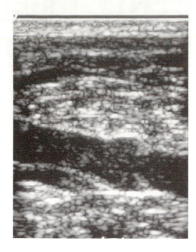

Gray scale image demonstrating a venous valve. (Courtesy of ATL, Bothell, Washington.)

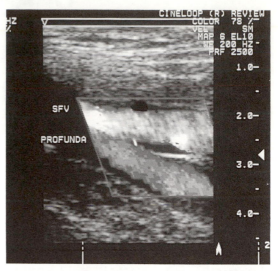

Color flow Doppler image at the level of the SFV and profunda vein insertions. See Color Plate 10 at the back of this book. (Courtesy of ATL, Bothell, Washington.)

PATIENT PREP

- None.

TRANSDUCER

- 5.0- or 7.0-MHz linear array with Doppler and/or color Doppler capabilities.

NORMAL SONOGRAPHIC FINDINGS

- There are five normal findings in duplex sonography of the lower extremity venous system.

  - Spontaneous flow: flow should be demonstrated with Doppler examination of the vessel immediately. A lack of flow may suggest thrombosis or external compression.

  - Phasicity: Doppler flow patterns vary because of the patient's respiratory changes:
    There will be a decrease in flow during inspiration due to increased intraabdominal pressure.
    Flow will increase with expiration.
    Continuous flow with no noticeable respiratory changes suggest a proximal obstruction.

  - Augmentation: with distal compression there should be a sudden rush of venous flow superiorly. This indicates no complete thrombosis between the transducer and the point of compression.

NOTE: If you need to compress a vein a second time to assess augmentation, you will need to wait a few seconds between compressions to allow the vein to refill distally.

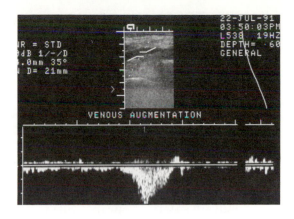

Spectral analysis image demonstrating venous augmentation. (Courtesy of Mary Washington Hospital, Fredericksburg, Virginia.)

– Competence of venous valves: there should be no venous blood flow in an inferior direction because of the presence of valves.

If you are sampling at a point inferior to a valve and the leg is compressed superior to the valve there should be no back flow of blood flow visible at the level of the transducer.

A valsalva maneuver may also be used to assess valve competence.

Any flow visible at the transducer with proximal compression represents incompetent valves. This may be due to old clot, which leaves the valves stiff and nonpliable, or varicose veins.

– Nonpulsatility: there are flow variations with respiratory cycles, not with each heartbeat.

NOTE: Pulsatile venous flow suggests congestive heart failure, fluid overload, or tricuspid insufficiency.

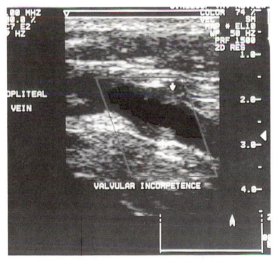

Color Doppler image demonstrating valvular incompetence. See Color Plate 11 at the back of this book. (Courtesy of ATL, Bothell, Washington.)

EXAM PROTOCOL AND REQUIRED IMAGES

NOTE: Examination of veins is easiest in a transverse plane, but longitudinal imaging should also be performed to help ensure adequate venous mapping (so that no small thrombosis is missed) and assessment of the venous valves especially with color flow Doppler.

We examine the veins transversely and then examine them longitudinally. We often rotate the probe as we go along to obtain the most information possible.

NOTE: Since a venous duplex examination requires a thorough mapping of the veins, it is unnecessary to perform a "survey" and then a more detailed exam to obtain images.

Images may be obtained as you go.

A built-in safety at our institution is that the radiologists quickly rescan all venous patients before they leave the department.

A diagnosis is rarely made from hard copy alone in this exam.

NOTE: Always examine both legs for comparative purposes. We find examining the asymptomatic leg first most helpful.

1. BEGIN TRANSVERSELY HIGH ON THE THIGH AT OR ABOVE THE LEVEL OF THE GROIN CREASE. LOCATE THE CFV AND CFA.

   TO CONFIRM THAT YOU ARE IN THE CFV, SCAN SLIGHTLY INFERIOR AND IDENTIFY THE SFV AND SAPHENOUS VEIN INSERTIONS. SUPERIOR TO THIS LEVEL IS THE CFV.

2. ASSESS THE ENTIRE LENGTH OF CFV VISIBLE FOR COMPRESSIBILITY BY COMPRESSING EVERY 1 TO 2 CM. THE CFA WILL NOT COMPRESS.

DOCUMENT IMAGE: ON A SPLIT SCREEN IF AVAILABLE

LT SCREEN: NONCOMPRESSED VEIN

RT SCREEN: COMPRESSED VEIN

LABELED: LT OR RT CFV

3. STILL AT THE LEVEL OF THE CFV TURN ON THE DOPPLER PLACING THE CURSOR TOWARD FLOW (WHEN USING THE DOPPLER FROM A TRANSVERSE PLANE, THE CURSOR SHOULD REMAIN PERPENDICULAR TO THE PROBE).

   SPONTANEOUS, PHASIC FLOW SHOULD BE PRESENT THROUGHOUT THE CFV.

DOCUMENT IMAGE: DUPLEX IMAGE WITH A SPECTRAL ANALYSIS OF CFV WAVEFORM DEMONSTRATING RESPIRATORY CHANGES

LABELED: RT OR LT CFV

4. RETURN TO A GRAY SCALE IMAGE (WE KEEP OUR DOPPLER CURSOR ON THE SCREEN OFF TO THE SIDE.) MOVE INFERIORLY AND LOCATE THE INSERTION OF THE SAPHENOUS VEIN MEDIALLY.

NOTE: Unless the saphenous vein is of greatest interest or pathology is suspected, we generally assess only the proximal portion of this vein. If necessary, the saphenous vein can easily be followed inferiorly along the medial aspect of the thigh and down the calf.

ASSESS THE PROXIMAL PORTION OF THE SAPHENOUS VEIN FOR COMPRESSIBILITY.

DOCUMENT IMAGE: ON A SPLIT SCREEN

LT SCREEN: NONCOMPRESSED VEIN

RT SCREEN: COMPRESSED VEIN

LABELED: RT OR LT SAPH V

5. INVESTIGATE THE PROXIMAL SEGMENT OF THE SAPHENOUS VEIN WITH DOPPLER. ASSESS FOR NORMAL CHARACTERISTICS.

DOCUMENT IMAGE: DUPLEX IMAGE OF A SPECTRAL ANALYSIS WAVEFORM FROM THE SAPHENOUS VEIN DEMONSTRATING AUGMENTATION OR RESPIRATORY CHANGES

LABELED: RT OR LT SAPH V

6. RETURN TO GRAY SCALE IMAGING AND RETURN TO THE LEVEL OF THE CFV. MOVE INFERIORLY TO LOCATE THE INSERTION OF THE PROFUNDA VEIN. THIS LIES POSTERIOR AND LATERAL TO THE SFV. FOLLOW THIS VEIN AS INFERIORLY AS POSSIBLE ASSESSING COMPRESSIBILITY.

NOTE: Compressibility may be difficult to assess in deep-lying vessels.

DOCUMENT IMAGE: SPLIT SCREEN

LT SCREEN: NONCOMPRESSED VEIN

RT SCREEN: COMPRESSED VEIN

LABELED: RT OR LT PROF V

7. RETURN SUPERIORLY TO THE DEEP VEIN INSERTION AND BEGIN SAMPLING WITH DOPPLER. ASSESS FOR NORMAL CHARACTERISTICS. FOLLOW AS INFERIORLY AS POSSIBLE.

NOTE: Generally, we document our images from the profunda vein close to its insertion where they are seen best.

DOCUMENT IMAGE: DUPLEX IMAGE OF A SPECTRAL ANALYSIS WAVEFORM FROM THE PROFUNDA VEIN DEMONSTRATING AUGMENTATION OR RESPIRATORY CHANGES

LABELED: RT OR LT PROF V

8. RETURN TO A GRAY SCALE IMAGE AND MOVE SUPERIOR TO THE LEVEL OF THE SFV INSERTION. BEGIN FOLLOWING THAT VEIN INFERIORLY COMPRESSING EVERY 1 TO 2 CM AT A LEVEL NEAR ITS INSERTION.

DOCUMENT IMAGE: SPLIT SCREEN

LT SCREEN: NONCOMPRESSED VEIN

RT SCREEN: COMPRESSED VEIN

LABELED: RT OR LT SFV

9. BEGIN TO SAMPLE THE SAME SEGMENT OF VEIN WITH DOPPLER. ASSESS FOR NORMAL CHARACTERISTICS.

DOCUMENT IMAGE: DUPLEX IMAGE OF A SPECTRAL ANALYSIS WAVEFORM FROM THE SFV NEAR ITS INSERTION DEMONSTRATING AUGMENTATION OR RESPIRATORY CHANGES

LABELED: RT OR LT SFV

10. RETURN TO A GRAY SCALE IMAGE AND CONTINUE TO FOLLOW THE SFV INFERIORLY ASSESSING FOR COMPRESSIBILITY.

NOTE: We make very careful note of vein compressibility because that is the most important indicator of venous thrombosis.

We often only sample with Doppler in the SFV at its insertion, midthigh, and most inferiorly. At each level we assess phasicity and augmentation.

AT APPROXIMATELY MIDTHIGH:

DOCUMENT IMAGE: SPLIT SCREEN

LT SCREEN: NONCOMPRESSED VEIN

RT SCREEN: COMPRESSED VEIN

LABELED: RT OR LT SFV MID

11. SAMPLE SFV AT A MIDTHIGH LEVEL WITH DOPPLER. ASSESS FOR NORMAL CHARACTERISTICS.

DOCUMENT IMAGE: DUPLEX IMAGE OF A SPECTRAL ANALYSIS WAVEFORM FROM THE SFV AT MIDTHIGH LEVEL DEMONSTRATING AUGMENTATION OR RESPIRATORY CHANGES

LABELED: RT OR LT SFV MID

12. RETURN TO A GRAY SCALE IMAGE AND INVESTIGATE THE REMAINING SEGMENT OF SFV, COMPRESSING AT REGULAR INTERVALS.

NOTE: As you approach Hunter's canal just superior to the knee, compression is often very difficult if possible at all. This is due to the tendons present here.

AS INFERIORLY AS POSSIBLE IN THE SFV:

DOCUMENT IMAGE: SPLIT SCREEN

LT SCREEN: NONCOMPRESSED VEIN

RT SCREEN: COMPRESSED VEIN

LABELED: RT OR LT SFV LOW OR INF

13. DOPPLER IN THE SFV JUST SUPERIOR TO THE KNEE. THE VEIN WILL HAVE PASSED MEDIALLY AND NOW LIES POSTERIOR TO THE ARTERY.

AUGMENTATION IS ESPECIALLY IMPORTANT HERE BECAUSE COMPRESSION IS OFTEN LESS THAN ADEQUATE.

DOCUMENT IMAGE: DUPLEX IMAGE OF A SPECTRAL ANALYSIS WAVEFORM FROM THE SFV JUST SUPERIOR TO THE KNEE DEMONSTRATING AUGMENTATION

LABELED: RT OR LT SFV LOW OR INF

14. THE POPLITEAL VEINS CAN BE EXAMINED EITHER WITH THE PATIENT PRONE OR WITH THE KNEE BENT AND RELAXED AWAY FROM THE PATIENT TO THE SIDE.

NOTE: Any vessel duplication, which is fairly common at this level. If there is more than one popliteal vessel they must both be carefully examined.

LOCATE THE POPLITEAL VEIN POSTERIOR TO THE ARTERY AND ASSESS FOR NORMAL CHARACTERISTICS.

FOLLOW THE VEIN AS FAR SUPERIORLY BEHIND THE THIGH AS POSSIBLE. CONTINUE TO ASSESS COMPRESSION.

BEGIN TO MOVE INFERIORLY, FOLLOWING THE POPLITEAL VEIN TO THE LEVEL OF ITS TRIFURCATION INTO THE CALF VEINS. FOLLOW THE POSTERIOR TIBIAL TRIBUTARY (THE LARGEST) AS FAR INFERIORLY AS POSSIBLE.

ONCE THE ENTIRE LENGTH OF THE POPLITEAL VEIN HAS BEEN ADEQUATELY ASSESSED FOR COMPRESSIBILITY, RETURN TO A MIDPOPLITEAL LEVEL.

DOCUMENT IMAGE: SPLIT SCREEN

LT SCREEN: NONCOMPRESSED VEIN

RT SCREEN: COMPRESSED VEIN

LABELED: RT OR LT POP V

15. WE OFTEN USE THE DOPPLER THROUGH THE ENTIRE LENGTH OF THE POPLITEAL VESSELS (OR USE COLOR DOPPLER). AT MIDPOPLITEAL LEVEL:

DOCUMENT IMAGE: DUPLEX IMAGE OF A SPECTRAL ANALYSIS WAVEFORM FROM THE MIDPOPLITEAL VEIN DEMONSTRATING AUGMENTATION

LABELED: RT OR LT POP V

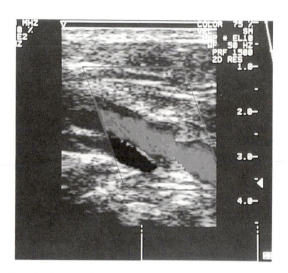

Color Doppler image of popliteal vein and artery. (See Color Plate 12 at the back of this book. (Courtesy of ATL, Bothell, Washington.)

NOTE: It may be awkward to squeeze a patient's thigh and maintain transducer location at the same time. Having the patient quickly flex the ipsilateral foot will have a similar effect.

16. IF COLOR DOPPLER IS AVAILABLE WE QUICKLY RESCAN THE ENTIRE LEG IN A LONGITUDINAL PLANE.

    COLOR DOPPLER PROVIDES A VISUAL MEANS OF ASSESSING SPONTANEOUS FLOW, AUGMENTATION, AND VALVE COMPETENCE.

17. TO ASSESS VALVE COMPETENCE WE RESCAN QUICKLY TO LOCATE A VENOUS VALVE (THIS MAY BE DONE WITHIN THE SCANNING PROTOCOL OF THAT PARTICULAR VENOUS SEGMENT) AND SCAN TO A LEVEL JUST INFERIOR TO THE VALVE.

    WHILE OBSERVING COLOR FLOW DOPPLER (OR A SPECTRAL ANALYSIS), SQUEEZE THE PATIENT'S LEG SUPERIOR TO THE VALVE. IF THE VALVE IS TOO SUPERIOR ALONG THE LEG, HAVE THE PATIENT TAKE IN A BREATH AND HOLD IT FOR A FEW SECONDS (VALSALVA MANEUVER).

    THERE SHOULD BE NO INFERIOR FLOW (BACK FLOW) OF VENOUS BLOOD THROUGH THE VALVE. REVERSE FLOW INDICATES THE PRESENCE OF AN INCOMPETENT VALVE.

    ANY VALVE CAN BE EXAMINED IN THIS MANNER.

18. AT OUR INSTITUTION WE EXAMINE ONLY THE DEEP VEINS OF THE THIGH. CALF VEINS CAN CERTAINLY BE EXAMINED FAIRLY EASILY, BUT THIS WILL NOT BE DISCUSSED AT THIS TIME.

    THE THEORY BEHIND EXAMINING ONLY THIGH VEINS IS THAT THESE ARE THE VEINS THAT PRODUCE LIFE-THREATENING PULMONARY EMBOLISM. THERE IS A SMALL INCIDENCE OF PULMONARY EMBOLISM DIRECTLY FROM CALF VEINS, BUT THE RISK IS MUCH SMALLER. THIS ISSUE IS STILL DEBATED CURRENTLY.

19. REPEAT ON THE AFFECTED LEG.

PATHOLOGY

Noncompressible Veins

● Clot: the vein lumen is generally enlarged compared with the opposite leg and usually contains some internal low to medium echoes.

Flow may be present if recanalization (reopening of the lumen) has begun.

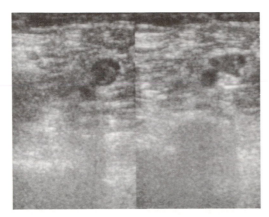

Split screen of clot-filled vein. Note small residual or recanalized lumen. (Courtesy of Mary Washington Hospital, Fredericksburg, Virginia.)

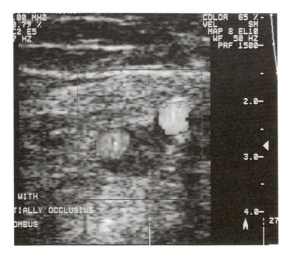

Color Doppler image demonstrating thrombus in the SFV. See Color Plate 13 at the back of this book. (Courtesy of ATL, Bothell, Washington.)

- Proximal obstruction: venous flow may be decreased and/or continuous.
  There are often no respiratory changes seen.
  The size of the vein may increase.

- Old clot: there are scarring changes present after an episode of venous thrombosis.
  There may be wall thickening, which may prevent complete compressibility.
  Be aware of the patient's history.
  Previous thrombosis may also affect the valve competence. Assess carefully.

Baker's Cyst

- A loculated fluid collection behind the knee (usually laterally) may cause leg swelling resulting from compression of the popliteal vein and associated poor venous drainage.

Cellulitis

- General inflammation of the skin and interstitial tissues of the leg. This most often affects the ankle and calf.
  The legs are often red and shiny.
  The deep veins may be more difficult to visualize because of the inflammation present.
  There is often increased echogenicity of the inflamed tissues, which may obscure vein visualization.

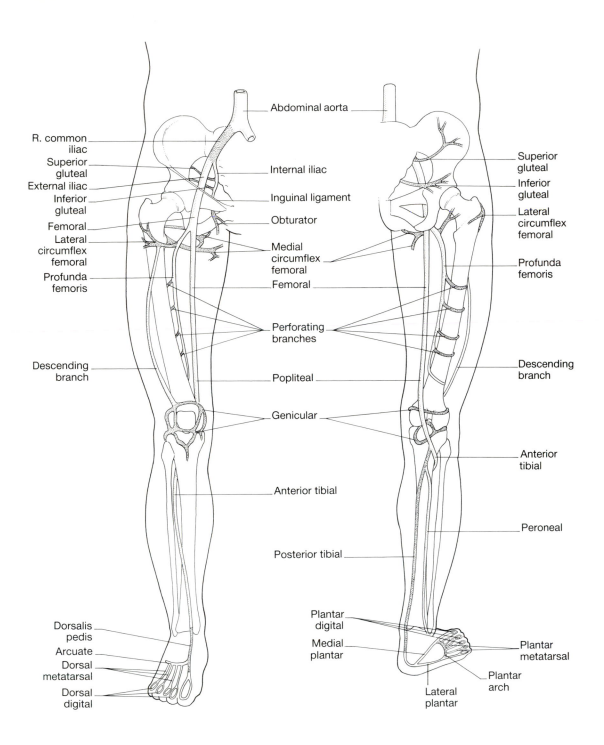

ARTERIAL SYSTEM OF
THE LOWER LIMB

Normal arterial anatomy of the legs.

LOWER EXTREMITY PERIPHERAL ARTERIAL DUPLEX ULTRASONOGRAPHY

- Purpose: to noninvasively determine the presence, amount, and location of arterial disease and plaque accumulation in the legs.

  - To assess claudication (cramping mainly behind the calf of the leg after exercise. This occurs because of an increased need for blood in the large muscle groups of the leg after exercise but a decreased available blood supply because of disease).

  - To assess graft patency (no blood pressures should be taken over or very close to a graft site. This could cause a leakage of blood at an anastomosis).

ANATOMY

PATIENT PREP

- None.

TRANSDUCER

- 5.0- or 7.0-MHz linear probe with Doppler and/or color Doppler capabilities. A 3.0-MHz probe is also helpful to examine the distal aorta and proximal iliac arteries.

NECESSARY EQUIPMENT

- Arm blood pressure cuff.
- Adult thigh blood pressure cuff.

EXAM PROTOCOL AND REQUIRED IMAGES

1. BEGINNING WITH THE PATIENT IN A SUPINE OR SITTING POSITION, OBTAIN BILATERAL BRACHIAL BLOOD PRESSURES. RECORD ON WORKSHEET (SEE SECTION ON BLOOD PRESSURES). PALPATE THE ULNAR AND RADIAL PULSES.

    PULSES SHOULD BE GRADED IN THE FOLLOWING MANNER:
    ++ BOUNDING
    + PALPABLE BUT FAINT
    0 NONPALPABLE

2. WITH THE PATIENT IN SUPINE POSITION, PALPATE THE FOLLOWING PULSES:
    GROIN (ILIAC/COMMON FEMORAL ARTERY)
    POPLITEAL
    POSTERIOR TIBIAL
    DORSALIS PEDIS

3. USING A 3.0-MHZ PROBE (OR A 5.0-MHZ PROBE ON A VERY THIN PATIENT), THE DISTAL AORTA AND PROXIMAL ILIAC ARTERIES SHOULD BE EXAMINED IN BOTH LONGITUDINAL AND TRANSVERSE PLANES.

    IMAGE: LONGITUDINAL DISTAL AORTA

    IMAGE: LONGITUDINAL RT ILIAC

    IMAGE: LONGITUDINAL LT ILIAC

NOTE: The iliac arteries may be examined simultaneously from a coronal longitudinal plane with the patient in a right lateral decubitus position.

IMAGE: TRANSVERSE DISTAL AORTA

IMAGE: TRANSVERSE RT/LT ILIAC ARTERY

NOTE: If one leg is significantly more symptomatic than the other, begin with the less symptomatic leg.

4. BEGIN SCANNING WITH A 5.0- OR 7.0-MHZ TRANSDUCER. YOU WILL NEED TO START SUPERIOR TO THE GROIN CREASE IN A SAGITTAL PLANE. LOCATE THE COMMON FEMORAL ARTERY (CFA).

5. SAMPLE WITH DOPPLER THOROUGHLY TO ASSESS BLOOD VELOCITIES AND PHASICITY THROUGHOUT THE LENGTH OF THE CFA.

    USE A CONTINUOUS DUPLEX MODE FOR ALL DUPLEX SAMPLING IF AVAILABLE. THIS MAKES SCANNING MUCH QUICKER.

NOTE: If a continuous duplex mode is not available, you will have to B-scan for a short segment, freeze an image, then move a Doppler cursor thoroughly over that frozen image, and continue on to the next segment through the entire vessel.

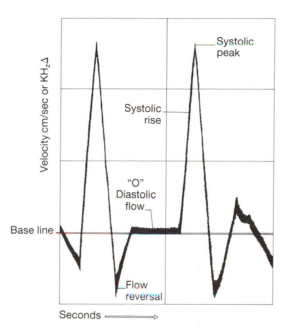

Normal triphasic arterial signal from a high-resistance system.

IMAGE: LONGITUDINAL GRAY SCALE (OR COLOR FLOW MAPPING) IMAGE OF THE CFA

LABELED: LONG RT OR LT CFA

IMAGE: DUPLEX SPECTRAL ANALYSIS OF THE CFA

LABELED: RT OR LT CFA

6. THE CFA WILL BIFURCATE INTO THE SUPERFICIAL FEMORAL ARTERY (SFA) AND THE DEEP FEMORAL OR PROFUNDA ARTERY.

7. FOLLOW THE PROFUNDA ARTERY AS INFERIORLY AS POSSIBLE WITH DUPLEX SAMPLING.

IMAGE: LONGITUDINAL VIEW OF THE PROFUNDA ARTERY ORIGIN

LABELED: RT OR LT PROF ART

IMAGE: DUPLEX SPECTRAL ANALYSIS OF THE PROFUNDA ARTERY NEAR ITS INSERTION

LABELED: RT OR LT PROF ART

NOTE: It may be difficult to follow the profunda for more than a few centimeters because the vessel usually courses deep into the leg. If you are able to follow the profunda artery for a longer length, another set of images should be documented more inferiorly along the vessel.

8. RETURN SUPERIORLY TO THE LEVEL OF THE BIFURCATION AND LOCATE THE SFA. FOLLOW THIS ARTERY INFERIORLY TO JUST ABOVE THE KNEE.

IMAGE: LONGITUDINAL VIEW OF THE SFA AT APPROXIMATELY MIDTHIGH

LABELED: RT OR LT MID SFA

IMAGE: DUPLEX SPECTRAL ANALYSIS AT MID THIGH

LABELED: RT OR LT MID SFA

IMAGE: LONGITUDINAL VIEW OF THE SFA JUST SUPERIOR TO THE KNEE

LABELED: RT OR LT DIST SFA

IMAGE: DUPLEX SPECTRAL ANALYSIS JUST SUPERIOR TO KNEE SFA

LABELED: RT OR LT DIST SFA

9. NEXT THE POPLITEAL ARTERY IS TO BE EXAMINED. THIS MAY BE DONE IN ONE OF TWO WAYS. EITHER THE PATIENT MAY BE PLACED IN A PRONE POSITION OR THE LEG MAY BE BENT SLIGHTLY AND RELAXED OUT TO THE SIDE AWAY FROM THE PATIENT.

PLACING THE PATIENT IN A PRONE POSITION WILL ALLOW FOR A MORE DIRECT, EASIER APPROACH, BUT IT MAY BE DIFFICULT OR TIME-CONSUMING TO HAVE THE PATIENT ROLL OVER.

10. LOCATE THE POPLITEAL ARTERY POSTERIOR AND SLIGHTLY LATERAL TO THE VEIN.

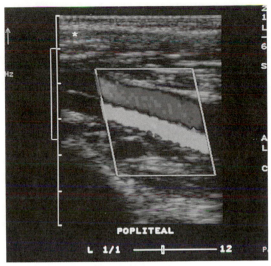

Color Doppler image of the popliteal artery. See Color Plate 14 at the back of this book. (Courtesy of Diasonics, Inc., Milpitas, California.)

FOLLOW THE ARTERY AS SUPERIORLY AS POSSIBLE INTO THE THIGH WHILE GRAY SCALE IMAGING.

BEGIN DUPLEX SAMPLING AND FOLLOW THE ARTERY AS INFERIORLY AS POSSIBLE TO THE SUPERIOR ASPECT OF THE CALF AT THE LEVEL OF THAT VESSEL'S BIFURCATION INTO THE TIBIOPERONEAL TRUNK AND THE ANTERIOR TIBIAL ARTERY.

IMAGE: LONGITUDINAL VIEW OF THE POPLITEAL ARTERY

LABELED: RT OR LT POP ART

IMAGE: DUPLEX SPECTRAL ANALYSIS OF THE POPLITEAL ARTERY

LABELED: RT OR LT POP ART

11. WE DO NOT FOLLOW THE INDIVIDUAL CALF ARTERIES DOWN THE THIGH, BUT THEY CAN BE MAPPED ESPECIALLY EASILY USING COLOR DOPPLER.

IT MAY BE HELPFUL TO FOLLOW THE ARTERIES UP THE LEG FROM THE ANKLE IF THERE IS ANY DIFFICULTY FOLLOWING THEM DOWN THE CALF.

12. AFTER EXAMINING THE POPLITEAL ARTERY, WE MOVE DOWN TO THE PATIENT'S ANKLE TO EXAMINE THE POSTERIOR TIBIAL ARTERY (PT) AND DORSALIS PEDIS ARTERY (DP).

BOTH ARTERIES SHOULD BE SAMPLED WITH DOPPLER. THE ARTERIES ARE OFTEN VERY SMALL, SO THE HIGHEST FREQUENCY TRANSDUCER AVAILABLE IS BEST.

NOTE: Gray scale images may be taken, but with these small vessels we do not take them as separate images unless some pathology is seen.

IMAGE: DUPLEX SPECTRAL ANALYSIS OF THE PT ARTERY

LABELED: RT OR LT PT

IMAGE: DUPLEX SPECTRAL ANALYSIS OF THE DP ARTERY

LABELED: RT OR LT DP

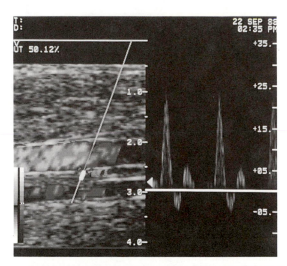

Spectral analysis of the posterior artery demonstrating normal triphasic flow. See Color Plate 15 at the back of this book. (Courtesy of ATL, Bothell, Washington.)

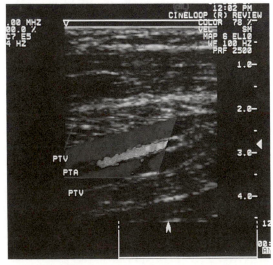

Color flow Doppler image of the posterior tibial artery and vein. See Color Plate 16 at the back of this book. (Courtesy of ATL, Bothell, Washington.)

NOTE: Determine the strongest and most easily accessible artery to use for pressure monitoring.

NOTE: The peroneal artery should also be examined at the ankle but rarely has a strong enough signal to be used for pressure monitoring.

NOTE: If a strong peroneal signal is present, a careful search for disease or occlusion in one of the other calf veins should be undertaken.

13. NOW THAT ALL VESSELS HAVE BEEN ASSESSED FOR PHASICITY AND VELOCITIES, WE MAY BEGIN TAKING THE BLOOD PRESSURES. CUFF PLACEMENT DEPENDS ON HOW MANY ARE AVAILABLE. CUFFS ARE TO BE PLACED AS FOLLOWS:
    AS HIGH AS POSSIBLE ON THE THIGH.
    JUST ABOVE THE KNEE.
    JUST BELOW THE KNEE.
    JUST ABOVE THE ANKLE.

14. IF ONLY ONE CUFF IS AVAILABLE IT MUST BE MOVED AFTER EACH PRECEDING SEGMENTAL PRESSURE HAS BEEN TAKEN.

    AN ARM CUFF IS USUALLY FINE FOR THE CALF PRESSURES.

15. USE THE POPLITEAL SIGNAL TO OBTAIN THE THIGH PRESSURES. RECORD THE PRESSURES.

16. REPOSITION THE PROBE AT THE STRONGEST ANKLE SIGNAL OBTAINED TO DETERMINE CALF PRESSURES. RECORD THE PRESSURES.

17. BLOOD PRESSURES SHOULD BE TAKEN IN THE FOLLOWING MANNER:
    THE CUFF SHOULD BE INFLATED TO A LEVEL ABOVE WHICH NO FLOW IS PRESENT.
    SLOWLY RELEASE THE PRESSURE.
    RECORD THE PRESSURE AT WHICH THE ARTERIAL SIGNAL FIRST RETURNS.
    IF YOU ARE UNABLE TO READ A PRESSURE THE FIRST TIME, DEFLATE THE CUFF COMPLETELY BEFORE REINFLATING.
    A PARTIAL REINFLATION MAY LEAD TO FALSELY LOW PRESSURES.

18. REPEAT ON THE CONTRALATERAL LEG.

NOTE: It may be difficult to obtain a high thigh pressure on obese patients.

When arterial wall hardening is present (i.e., with diabetic patients), pressures may be falsely elevated (may exceed 300 mm Hg).

NOTE: The examination may begin at the level of the common femoral vein, excluding imaging of the aorta and common iliac veins.

Two blood pressures may be obtained on each leg instead of four. One will be taken at midthigh and one at midcalf:

This will adequately demonstrate any drop in blood pressure and, therefore, any significant disease.

This is often used as a screening test.

Some laboratories have forgone the use of any blood pressures:

Vessel phasicity and plaque visualization are used for diagnostic purposes instead.

DATA DOCUMENTATION

Using Blood Pressures

- The severity of atherosclerotic disease may be assessed by using the ankle/arm index.

A/A INDEX

>1.13	Arterial calcifications
+1.0	Normal
0.9–1.0	Minimal ischemia with minimal symptoms
0.5–0.9	Mild to moderate ischemia with mild to moderate claudication
0.3–0.5	Moderate to severe ischemia with severe claudication or rest pain
<0.3	Severe ischemia with rest pain or gangrene

- The A/A index must be calculated after all pressures have been taken and recorded.

NOTE: A general rule of thumb is that any segmental pressure drop of 20 mm Hg or more represents significant pathology.

Without Blood Pressures

- Phasicity.

  - Triphasic signals: have a strong forward systolic component followed by a brief period of diastolic flow reversal and then an end diastolic forward flow segment.
  This is due to the high resistance flow present in the legs.

  - Biphasic signals: have a strong forward systolic component followed by a period of diastolic flow reversal.
  There is no end diastolic forward flow component.

  - Monophasic signals: contain only systolic forward flow.

- Study interpretation.

  - Normal: all signals remain triphasic.

  - Mild disease: Spectral broadening with loss of spectral window. Signals biphasic.

  - Moderate disease: Systolic velocity elevation. Signals may remain biphasic.

  - Severe disease: Monophasic signals with elevated peak systolic velocities and spectral broadening.

MARY WASHINGTON HOSPITAL
PERIPHERAL ARTERIAL STUDY WORKSHEET

NAME: _____   DATE: _____

X RAY #: _____   DOCTOR: _____

AGE: _____

SYMPTOMS: _____

CLAUDICATION: R   L   DIABETES: Y   N   HYPERTENSION: Y   N

PULSES: RT   LT

RADIAL   _____   _____
ULNAR   _____   _____
FEMORAL   _____   _____
PT   _____   _____
DP   _____   _____

BLOOD PRESSURES: RT   LT

          BRACHIAL: _____   _____

RT A/A INDEX: RT CIA   LT CIA

                                       RT FEM A   LT FEM A
_____

                                       RT POP BP   LT POP BP

LT A/A INDEX: _____   _____

                                       RT PT   LT PT
_____   _____   _____

An example of a worksheet for a peripheral arterial examination utilizing blood pressure. (Courtesy of Mary Washington Hospital, Fredericksburg, Virginia.)

ABBREVIATION GLOSSARY

ANT: Anterior

BIF: Bifurcation

CBD: Common bile duct

CC: Cubic centimeter

CD: Common duct

CERX: Cervix

CHD: Common hepatic duct

Cm: Centimeter

COR: Coronal

CR: Crown rump

C-SPINE: Cervical spine

DECUB: Decubitus

ER: Endorectal

EV: Endovaginal

GB: Gallbladder

GS: Gestational sac

IN: Inches

INF: Inferior

IVC: Inferior vena cava

KID: Kidney

LAT: Lateral

LLD: Left lateral decubitus

LPO: Left posterior oblique

L-SPINE: Lumbar spine

LT: Left

MED: Medial

MHz: Megahertz

ML: Midline

Mm: Millimeter

NIP: Nipple

OBL: Oblique

OV: Ovary

POP: Popliteal artery

POST: Posterior

PROX: Proximal

RLD: Right lateral decubitus

RPO: Right posterior oblique

RT: Right

SAG: Sagittal

SEM V: Seminal vesicles

SUP: Superior

TGC: Time-gain compensation

TRV: Transverse

T-SPINE: Thoracic spine

UT: Uterus

VAG: Vagina

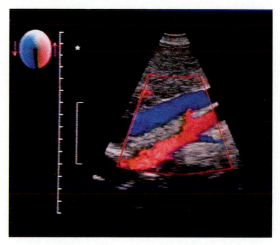

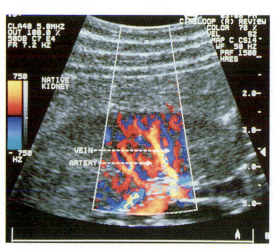

Plate 1. Color Doppler image demonstrating renal artery origins. (Courtesy of Diasonics, Inc., Milpitas, California.)

Plate 2. Color Doppler image demonstrating renal perfusion. (Courtesy of ATL, Bothell, Washington.)

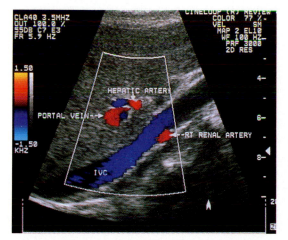

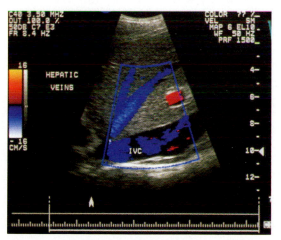

Plate 3. Color Doppler image demonstrating flow in the region of the porta hepatis. (Courtesy of ATL, Bothell, Washington.)

Plate 4. Example of color flow Doppler in hepatic veins. (Courtesy of ATL, Bothell, Washington.)

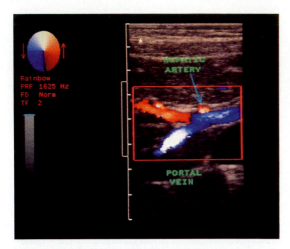

Plate 5. Example of color Doppler image of flow in the portal vein.

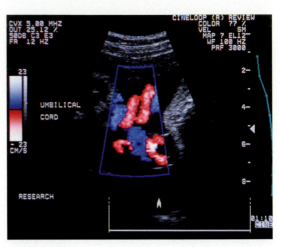

Plate 6. Color Doppler image of a three-vessel umbilical cord.

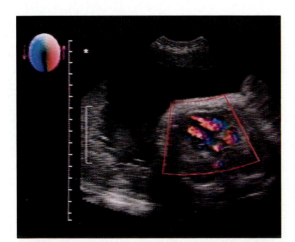

Plate 7. Color Doppler image of a fetal four-chamber heart. (Courtesy of Diasonics, Inc. Milpitas, California. Diasonics does not have the Food and Drug Administration approval to market their probes for this fetal Doppler application. However, the final decision as to how a medical device will be used is the prerogative of the medical practitioner. Please check FDA approval for all manufacturers' probes used in any examination.)

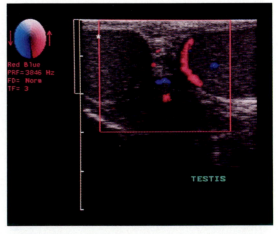

Plate 8. Color Doppler image demonstrating arterial flow in a testicular artery. (Courtesy of Diasonics, Inc., Milpitas, California.)

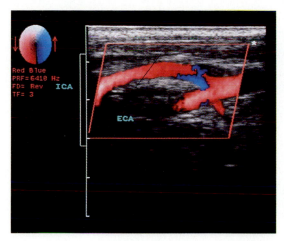

Plate 9. Color Doppler image of the carotid artery bifurcation. (Courtesy of Diasonics, Inc., Milpitas, California.)

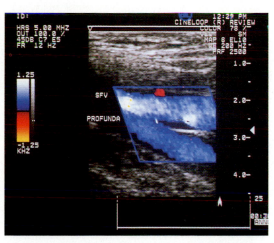

Plate 10. Color flow Doppler image at the level of the SFV and profunda vein insertions. (Courtesy of ATL, Bothell, Washington.)

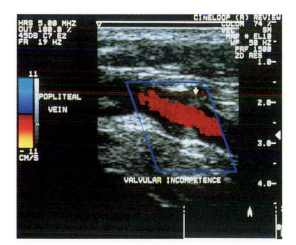

Plate 11. Color Doppler image demonstrating valvular incompetence. (Courtesy of ATL, Bothell, Washington.)

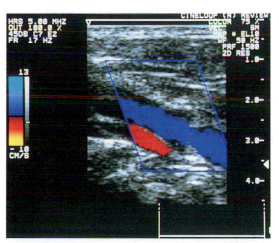

Plate 12. Color Doppler image of popliteal vein and artery. (Courtesy of ATL, Bothell, Washington.)

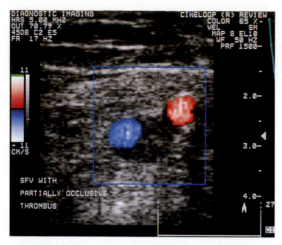

Plate 13. Color Doppler image demonstrating thrombus in the SFV. (Courtesy of ATL, Bothell, Washington.)

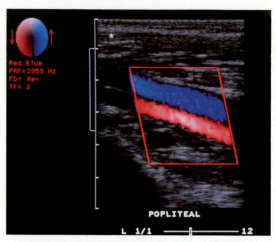

Plate 14. Color Doppler image of the popliteal artery. (Courtesy of Diasonics, Inc., Milpitas, California.)

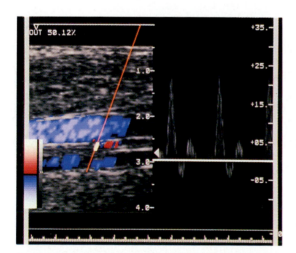

Plate 15. Spectral analysis of the posterior artery, demonstrating normal triphasic flow. (Courtesy of ATL, Bothell, Washington.)

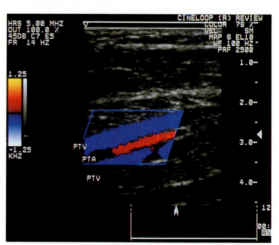

Plate 16. Color flow Doppler image of the posterior tibial artery and vein. (Courtesy of ATL, Bothell, Washington.)

GUIDELINES FOR PERFORMANCE OF THE ABDOMINAL AND RETROPERITONEAL ULTRASOUND EXAMINATION*

The following are proposed guidelines for ultrasound evaluation of the upper abdomen. The document consists of two parts:

Part I: Equipment and Documentation Guidelines
Part II: Guidelines for a General Examination of the Abdomen and Retroperitoneum

These guidelines have been developed to provide assistance to practitioners performing ultrasound studies in the abdomen and retroperitoneum. In some cases, additional and/or specialized examinations may be necessary. While it is not possible to detect every abnormality, adherence to the following guidelines will maximize the probability of detecting most of the abnormalities that occur in the abdomen and retroperitoneum.

PART I

GUIDELINES FOR EQUIPMENT AND DOCUMENTATION

Equipment

Abdominal and retroperitoneal studies should be conducted with a real-time scanner, preferably using sector or curved linear trans-

---

*From American Institute of Ultrasound in Medicine. Additional copies of guidelines can be ordered from the AIUM at the cost of $6.00 for AIUM members and $20.00 for nonmembers. Mail orders to AIUM Publications Department, 11200 Rockville Pike, Suite 205, Rockville MD 20852-3139.

ducers. Static B-scan images may be obtained as a supplement to the real-time images when indicated. The transducer or scanner should be adjusted to operate at the highest clinically appropriate frequency, realizing that there is a trade-off between resolution and beam penetration. With modern equipment, these frequencies are usually between 2.25 and 5.0 MHz.

Documentation

Adequate documentation is essential for high-quality patient care. This should be a permanent record of the ultrasound examination and its interpretation. Images of all appropriate areas, both normal and abnormal, should be recorded in appropriate imaging or storage format. Variations from normal size should be accompanied by measurements. Images are to be appropriately labeled with the examination date, patient identification, and image orientation. A report of the ultrasound findings should be included in the patient's medical record, regardless of where the study is performed. Retention of the ultrasound examination should be consistent both with clinical need and with relevant legal and local health care facility requirements.

PART II

GUIDELINES FOR THE ABDOMEN AND RETROPERITONEUM ULTRASOUND EXAMINATION

The following guidelines describe the examination to be performed for each organ and anatomical region in the abdomen and retroperitoneum. A complete examination would include all of the following. A limited examination would include only one or more of these areas, but not all of them.

Liver

The liver survey should include both long axis (coronal or sagittal) and transverse views. If possible, views comparing the echogenicity of the liver to the right kidney should be performed. The major vessels (aorta/inferior vena cava) in the region of the liver should be imaged, including the position of the inferior vena cava where it passes through the liver.

The regions of the ligamentum teres on the left and of the dome of the right lobe with the right hemidiaphragm and right pleural space should be imaged. The main lobar fissure should be demonstrated.

Survey of right and left lobes should include visualization of the hepatic veins. The right and left branches of the portal vein should be identified. The intrahepatic bile ducts should be evaluated for possible dilatation.

Gallbladder and Biliary Tract

The gallbladder evaluation should include long axis (coronal or sagittal) and transverse views obtained in the supine position. Left lateral decubitus (left side down), erect, or prone positions may also be necessary to allow a complete evaluation of the gallbladder and its surrounding area.

The intrahepatic ducts can be evaluated, as described under the liver, by obtaining views of the liver demonstrating the right and left hepatic branches of the portal vein. The extrahepatic ducts can be evaluated in supine, left lateral decubitus, and/or semierect positions. The size of the intrahepatic and extrahepatic ducts should be assessed. With these views the relationship between the bile ducts, hepatic artery, and portal vein can be shown. When possible, the common bile duct in the pancreatic head should be visualized.

Pancreas

The pancreatic head, uncinate process, and body should be identified in transverse, and, when possible, long axis (coronal or sagittal) projections. If possible, the pancreatic tail should also be imaged, and the pancreatic duct demonstrated. The peripancreatic region should be assessed for adenopathy.

Spleen

Representative views of the spleen in long axis, either sagittal or coronal, and in transverse projection should be performed. An attempt should be made to demonstrate the left pleural space. When possible, the echogenicity of the upper pole of the left kidney should be compared to that of the spleen.

Kidneys

Representative long axis (coronal or sagittal) views of each kidney should be obtained, visualizing the cortex and the renal pelvis. Transverse views of both the left and right kidney should include the upper pole, middle section at the renal pelvis, and the lower pole. When possible, comparison of renal echogenicity with the adjacent liver and spleen should be performed. The perirenal regions should be assessed for possible abnormality.

Aorta and Inferior Vena Cava

The aorta and inferior vena cava should be imaged in long axis (either sagittal or coronal) and transverse planes. Scans of both vessels should be attempted from the diaphragm to the bifurcation (usually at the level of the umbilicus). If possible, images should also include the adjacent common iliac vessels.

Abnormalities should be assessed. The surrounding soft tissues should be evaluated for adenopathy.

GUIDELINES FOR PERFORMANCE OF THE SCROTAL ULTRASOUND EXAMINATION*

The following are proposed guidelines for ultrasound evaluation of the scrotum. The document consists of two parts:

Part I: Equipment and Documentation Guidelines
Part II: Guidelines for a General Examination of the Scrotum

These guidelines have been developed to provide assistance to practitioners performing ultrasound studies in the scrotum. In some cases, additional and/or specialized examinations may be necessary. While it is not possible to detect every abnormality, adherence to the following guidelines will maximize the probability of detecting most of the abnormalities that occur in the scrotum.

PART I

GUIDELINES FOR EQUIPMENT AND DOCUMENTATION

Equipment

Scrotal studies should be conducted with a real-time scanner, preferably using sector or curved linear transducers. Static B-scan images may be obtained as a supplement to the real-time images when indicated. The transducer or scanner should be adjusted to operate at the highest clinically appropriate frequency, realizing that there is a trade-off between resolution and beam penetration. With

---

*From American Institute of Ultrasound in Medicine. Additional copies of guidelines can be ordered from the AIUM at the cost of $6.00 for AIUM members and $20.00 for nonmembers. Mail orders to AIUM Publications Department, 11200 Rockville Pike, Suite 205, Rockville, MD 20852-3139.

modern equipment, these frequencies are usually between 2.25 and 5.0 MHz or greater.

COMMENT: Resolution should be of sufficient quality to routinely differentiate small cystic from solid lesions.

Documentation

Adequate documentation is essential for high-quality patient care. This should be a permanent record of the ultrasound examination and its interpretation. Images of all appropriate areas, both normal and abnormal, should be recorded in any image format. Variations from normal size should be accompanied by measurements. Images are to be appropriately labeled with the examination date, patient identification, and image orientation. A report of the ultrasound findings should be included in the patient's medical record, regardless of where the study is performed. Retention of the ultrasound examination should be consistent both with clinical need and with relevant legal and local health care facility requirements.

PART II

GUIDELINES FOR THE SCROTAL ULTRASOUND EXAMINATION

The testes should be studied in at least two projections, long axis and transverse. Views of each testicle should include the superior, mid, and inferior portions as well as its medial and lateral borders. The adjacent epididymis should be evaluated. The size and echogenicity of each testicle and epididymis should be compared to its opposite side.

Any abnormality should be documented and all extratesticular structures evaluated. Additional techniques such as Valsalva maneuver or upright positioning can be utilized as needed.

APPENDIX III
GUIDELINES FOR PERFORMANCE OF THE ANTEPARTUM OBSTETRICAL ULTRASOUND EXAMINATION*

These guidelines have been developed for use by practitioners performing obstetrical ultrasound studies. A limited examination may be performed in clinical emergencies or if used as a follow-up to a complete examination. In some cases, an additional and/or specialized examination may be necessary. While it is not possible to detect all structural congenital anomalies with diagnostic ultrasound, adherence to the following guidelines will maximize the possibility of detecting many fetal abnormalities.

EQUIPMENT

These studies should be conducted with real-time scanners, using an abdominal and/or vaginal approach. A transducer of appropriate frequency (3 MHz or higher abdominally, 5 MHz or higher vaginally) should be used. A static scanner (3 to 5 MHz) may be used but should not be the sole method of examination. The lowest possible ultrasonic exposure settings should be used to gain the necessary diagnostic information.

> *COMMENT:* Real-time is necessary to reliably confirm the presence of fetal life through observation of cardiac activity, respiration, and active movement. Real-time studies simplify evaluation of fetal anatomy as well as the task of obtaining fetal measurements. The choice of frequency is a trade-off be-

*From American Institute of Ultrasound in Medicine. Additional copies of guidelines can be ordered from the AIUM at the cost of $6.00 for AIUM members and $20.00 for nonmembers. Mail orders to AIUM Publications Department, 11200 Rockville Pike, Suite 205, Rockville, MD 20852-3139.

tween beam penetration and resolution. With modern equipment, 3- to 5-MHz abdominal transducers allow sufficient penetration in nearly all patients, while providing adequate resolution. During early pregnancy, a 5-MHz abdominal or a 5- to 7-MHz vaginal transducer may provide adequate penetration and produce superior resolution.

DOCUMENTATION

Adequate documentation of the study is essential for high-quality patient care. This should include a permanent record of the ultrasound images, incorporating whenever possible the measurement parameters and anatomical findings proposed in the following sections of this document. Images should be appropriately labeled with the examination date, patient identification, and, if appropriate, image orientation. A written report of the ultrasound findings should be included in the patient's medical record regardless of where the study is performed.

GUIDELINES FOR FIRST TRIMESTER SONOGRAPHY

Overall Comment: Scanning in the first trimester may be performed either abdominally or vaginally. If an abdominal scan is performed and fails to provide definitive information concerning any of the following guidelines, a vaginal scan should be performed whenever possible.

1. The location of the gestational sac should be documented. The embryo should be identified and the crown-rump length recorded.

   COMMENT: The crown-rump length is an accurate indicator of fetal age. Comparison should be made to standard tables. If the embryo is not identified, characteristics of the gestational sac including mean diameter of the anechoic space to determine fetal age and analysis of the hyperechoic rim should be noted. During the late first trimester, biparietal diameter and other fetal measurements may also be used to establish fetal age.

2. Presence or absence of fetal life should be reported.

   COMMENT: Real-time observation is critical in this diagnosis. It should be noted that fetal cardiac activity may not be visible prior to 7 weeks abdominally and frequently at least 1 week earlier vaginally as determined by crown-rump length. Thus, confirmation of fetal life may require follow-up evaluation.

3. Fetal number should be documented.

   COMMENT: Multiple pregnancies should be reported only in those instances where multiple embryos are seen. Due to variability in fusion between the amnion and chorion, the appearance of more than one sac-like structure in early pregnancy is often noted and may be confused with multiple gestation or amniotic band.

4. Evaluation of the uterus (including cervix) and adnexal structures should be performed.

   COMMENT: This will allow recognition of incidental findings of potential clinical significance. The presence, location, and size of myomas and adnexal masses should be recorded.

GUIDELINES FOR SECOND AND THIRD TRIMESTER SONOGRAPHY

1. Fetal life, number, and presentation should be documented.

   COMMENT: Abnormal heart rate and/or rhythm should be reported. Multiple pregnancies require the reporting of additional information: placental number, sac number, comparison of fetal size, and when visualized, fetal genitalia, and presence or absence of an interposed membrane.

2. An estimate of the amount of amniotic fluid (increased, decreased, normal) should be reported.

   COMMENT: While this evaluation is subjective, there is little difficulty in recognizing the extremes of amniotic fluid volume. Physiological variation with stage of pregnancy must be taken into account.

3. The placental location, appearance, and its relationship to the internal cervical os should be recorded.

   COMMENT: It is recognized that placental position early in pregnancy may not correlate well with its location at the time of delivery.

4. Assessment of gestational age should be accomplished using combination of biparietal diameter (or head circumference) and femur length. Fetal growth and weight (as opposed to age) should be assessed in the third trimester and requires the addition of abdominal diameters or circumferences. If previous studies have been performed, an estimate of the appropriateness of interval change should be given.

   COMMENT: Third trimester measurements may not accurately reflect gestational age. Initial determination of gestational age should therefore be performed prior to the third trimester whenever possible. If one or more previous studies have been performed, the gestational age at the time of the current examination should be based on the earliest examination that permits measurement of crown-rump length, biparietal diameter, head circumference, and/or femur length by the equation: current fetal age equals initial embryo/fetal age plus number of weeks from first study. The current measurements should be compared with norms for the gestational age based on standard tables. If previous studies have been performed, interval change in the measurements should be assessed.

4A. Biparietal diameter at a standard reference level (which should include the cavum septi pellucidi, and the thalamus) should be measured and recorded.

COMMENT: If the fetal head is dolichocephalic or brachycephalic, the biparietal diameter alone may be misleading. On occasion, the computation of the cephalic index, a ratio of the biparietal diameter to fronto-occipital diameter, is needed to make this determination. In such situations, the head circumference or corrected biparietal diameter is required.

4B. Head circumference is measured at the same level as the biparietal diameter.

4C. Femur length should be measured routinely and recorded after the 14th week of gestation.

COMMENT: As with biparietal diameter, considerable biological variation is present late in pregnancy.

4D. Abdominal circumference should be determined at the level of the junction of the umbilical vein and portal sinus.

COMMENT: Abdominal circumference measurement may allow detection of growth retardation and macrosomia—conditions of the late second and third trimester. Comparison of the abdominal circumference with the head circumference should be made. If the abdominal measurement is below or above that expected for a stated gestation, it is recommended that circumferences of the head and body be measured and the head circumference/abdominal circumference ratio be reported. The use of circumferences is also suggested in those instances where the shape of either the head or body is different from that normally encountered.

5. Evaluation of the uterus and adnexal structures should be performed.

COMMENT: This will allow recognition of incidental findings of potential clinical significance. The presence, location, and size of myomas and adnexal masses should be recorded.

6. The study should include, but not necessarily be limited to, the following fetal anatomy: cerebral ventricles, four-chamber view of the heart (including its position within the thorax), spine, stomach, urinary bladder, umbilical cord insertion site on the anterior abdominal wall, and renal region.

COMMENT: It is recognized that not all malformations of the above-mentioned organ systems (such as the spine) can be detected using ultrasonography. Nevertheless, a careful anatomical survey may allow diagnosis of certain birth defects which would otherwise go unrecognized. Suspected abnormalities may require a specialized evaluation.

GUIDELINES FOR PERFORMANCE OF THE ULTRASOUND EXAMINATION OF THE FEMALE PELVIS*

The following are proposed guidelines for ultrasound evaluation of the female pelvis. The document consists of two parts:

Part I: Equipment and Documentation Guidelines
Part II: Guidelines for the General Examination of the Female Pelvis

These guidelines have been developed to provide assistance to practitioners performing ultrasound studies of the female pelvis. In some cases, additional and/or specialized examinations may be necessary. While it is not possible to detect every abnormality, adherence to the following guidelines will maximize the probability of detecting most of the abnormalities that occur.

PART I

GUIDELINES FOR EQUIPMENT AND DOCUMENTATION

Equipment

Ultrasound examination of the female pelvis should be conducted with a real-time scanner, preferably using sector or curved linear transducers. Static B-scan images may be obtained as a supplement to the real-time images when indicated. The transducer or scanner should be adjusted to operate at the highest clinically appropriate frequency, realizing that there is a trade-off between resolution

*From American Institute of Ultrasound in Medicine. Additional copies of guidelines can be ordered from the AIUM at the cost of $6.00 for AIUM members and $20.00 for nonmembers. Mail orders to AIUM Publications Department, 11200 Rockville Pike, Suite 205, Rockville, MD 20852-3139.

and beam penetration. With modern equipment, studies performed from the anterior abdominal wall can usually use frequencies of 3.5 MHz or higher, while scans performed from the vagina should use frequencies of 5 MHz or higher.

Care of the Equipment

Vaginal probes should be covered by a protective sheath prior to insertion. Following the examination, the sheath should be disposed and the probe cleaned in an antimicrobial solution. The type of solution and amount of time for cleaning depends on manufacturer and infectious disease recommendations.

Documentation

Adequate documentation is essential for high quality patient care. There should be a permanent record of the ultrasound examination and its interpretation. Images of all appropriate areas, both normal and abnormal, should be recorded in an imaging or storage format. Variations from normal size should be accompanied by measurements. Images are to be appropriately labeled with the examination date, patient identification and image orientation. A report of the ultrasound findings should be included in the patient's medical record. Retention of the permanent record of the ultrasound examination should be consistent both with clinical need and with the relevant legal and local health care facility requirements.

PART II

GUIDELINES FOR PERFORMANCE OF THE ULTRASOUND EXAMINATION OF THE FEMALE PELVIS

The following guidelines describe the examination to be performed for each organ and anatomic region in the female pelvis. Identifying all relevant structures should be identified by the abdominal or vaginal approach, in some cases, both will be necessary.

General Pelvic Preparation

For a pelvic sonogram performed from the abdominal wall, the patient's urinary bladder should be filled. For a vaginal sonogram, the urinary bladder is usually empty. The vaginal transducer may be introduced by the patient, the sonographer, or the sonologist. It is recommended that a woman should be present in the examining room at all times during a vaginal sonogram, either as an examiner or a chaperone.

Uterus

The vagina and uterus provide an anatomic landmark that can be utilized as a reference point for the remaining normal and abnormal pelvic structures. In evaluating the uterus, the following should be documented: a) the uterine size, shape, and orientation; b) the endometrium; c) the myometrium; and d) the cervix. The vagina should be imaged as a landmark for the cervix and lower uterine segment.

Uterine size can be obtained. Uterine length is evaluated in long axis from the fundus to the cervix (the external os, if it can be identified). The depth of the uterus (anteroposterior dimension) is measured in the same long axis view from its anterior to posterior walls, perpendicular to the length. The width is measured from the transaxial or coronal view. Cervical diameters can be similarly obtained.

Abnormalities of the uterus should be documented. The endometrium should be analyzed for thickness, echogenicity and its position within the uterus. The myometrium and cervix should be evaluated for contour changes, echogenicity, and masses.

Adnexa (Ovaries and Fallopian Tubes)

When evaluating the adnexa, an attempt should be made to identify the ovaries first since they can serve as the major point of reference for adnexal structures. Frequently the ovaries are situated anterior to the internal iliac (hypogastric) vessels, which serve as a landmark for their identification. The following ovarian findings should be documented; a) size, shape, contour, and echogenicity and b) position relative to the uterus. The ovarian size can be determined by measuring the length in long axis, usually along the axis of the hypogastric (internal iliac) vessels, with the anteroposterior dimension measured perpendicular to the length. The ovarian width is measured in the transaxial or coronal view. A volume can be calculated.

The normal fallopian tubes are not commonly identified. This region should be surveyed for abnormalities, particularly dilated tubular structures.

If an adnexal mass is noted, its relationship to the ovaries and uterus should be documented. Its size and echopattern (cystic, solid or mixed) shold be determined.

Cul-de-Sac

The cul-de-sac and bowel posterior to the uterus may not be clearly defined. This area should be evaluated for the presence of free fluid or mass. If a mass is detected, its size, position, shape, echopattern (cystic, solid or complex), and its relationship to the ovaries and uterus should be documented. Differentiation of normal loops of bowel from a mass may be difficult if only an abdominal examination is performed. If a suspected mass is imaged that might represent fluid and feces within normal rectosigmoid colon and a vaginal scan is not performed, an ultrasound water enema study or a repeat examination after a cleansing enema may be indicated.

GUIDELINES FOR PERFORMANCE OF THE ULTRASOUND EXAMINATION OF THE PROSTATE (AND SURROUNDING STRUCTURES)*

The following are proposed guidelines for the ultrasound evaluation of the prostate and surrounding structures. The document consists of two parts:

Part I: Equipment and Documentation
Part II: Ultrasound Examination of the Prostate and Surrounding Structures

These guidelines have been developed to provide assistance to practitioners performing an ultrasound study of the prostate. In some cases, an additional and/or specialized examination may be necessary. While it is not possible to detect every abnormality, adherence to the following will maximize the detection of most abnormalities.

PART I

EQUIPMENT AND DOCUMENTATION

Equipment

A prostate study should be conducted with a real-time transrectal (also termed endorectal) transducer using the highest clinically ap-

---

*From American Institute of Ultrasound in Medicine. Additional copies of guidelines can be ordered from AIUM at the cost of $6.00 for AIUM members and $20.00 for nonmembers. Mail orders to AIUM Publications Department, 11200 Rockville Pike, Suite 205, Rockville, MD 20852-3139.

propriate frequency, realizing that there is a trade-off between resolution and beam penetration. With modern equipment, these frequencies are usually 5 MHz or higher.

Documentation

Adequate documentation is essential for high quality patient care. There should be a permanent record of the ultrasound examination and its interpretation. Images of all appropriate areas, both normal and abnormal, should be accompanied by measurements. Images are to be appropriately labeled with the examination date, patient identification, and image orientation. A report of the ultrasound findings should be included in the patient's medical record. Retention of the permanent record of the ultrasound examination should be consistent both with clinical need and with the relevant legal and local health care facility requirements.

Care of the Equipment

Transrectal probes should be covered by a disposable sheath prior to insertion. Following the examination, the sheath should be disposed, and the probe soaked in an antimicrobial solution. The type of solution and amount of time for soaking depends on manufacturer and infectious disease recommendations. Following the examination, if there is a gross tear in the sheath, the fluid channels in the probe should be thoroughly flushed with the antimicrobial solution. Tubing and stop cocks should be disposed after each examination.

PART II

ULTRASOUND EXAMINATION OF THE PROSTATE AND SURROUNDING STRUCTURES

The following guidelines describe the examination to be performed for the prostate and surrounding structures.

Prostate

The prostate should be imaged in its entirety in at least two orthogonal planes, sagittal and axial or sagittal and coronal, from the apex to the base of the gland. In particular, the peripheral zone should be thoroughly imaged. The gland should be evaluated for size, echogenicity, symmetry, and continuity of margins. The periprostatic fat and vessels should be evaluated for asymmetry and disruption in echogenicity.

Seminal Vesicles and Vas Deferens

The seminal vesicles should be examined in two planes from their insertion into the prostate via the ejaculatory ducts to their cranial and lateral extents. They should be evaluated for size, shape, position, symmetry, and echogenicity. Both vas deferens should be evaluated.

Perirectal Space

Evaluation of the perirectal space, in particular the region that abuts on the prostate and perirectal tissues, should be performed. If rectal pathology is clinically suspected, the rectal wall and lumen should be studied.

INDEX

Note: Page numbers in *italics* refer to illustrations. Numbers followed by t indicate tables.

325

35 #2
45 #5
73 #5
89 #4